Broccoli, Love & Dark Chocolate

BROCCOLI LOVE & DARK CHOCOLATE

Because food, love, and life should be delicious!

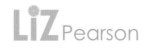

whitecap

For my two daughters, Chelsea and Shannon

EDITORS Theresa Best and Tracy Bordian
DESIGNER Setareh Ashrafologhalai
FOOD PHOTOGRAPHY Liz Pearson
ADDITIONAL PHOTOGRAPHY foodograph.ca (9, 63, 222); iStockphoto.com: dcdr (iii), SchulteProductions (v), jml5571 (3), morningarage (4), amandagrand (6), Jag_cz (8), greatideapl (11), jrwasserman (13), mariusFM77 (14), tanya_emsh (15), Elenathewise (17), jirkaejc (19), russlann (21), olgakr (22), tycoon751 (23), matka_Wariatka (25), tirc83 (29), LdF (31), loooby (33), GMVozd (35), isa-7777 (40), robynmac (43), egal (46), leeser87 (48), anthonyjhall (57), nsilcock (59), Shinyshot (67), ArturNyk (72), sematadesign (74), tashka2000 (84), Nanisimova (87), barol16 (89), minadezhda (92), intraprese (95), wholden (96), sf_foodphoto (98), ValentynVolkov (101), MurrayProductions (105), barol16 (107), annata78 (115), markos86 (116), andresrimaging (122), Teleginatania (129), dageldog (132), Zakharova_Natalia (135), IngaNielsen (138), 4774344sean (142), stevecoleimages (150), Studio1One (154), MistikaS (169), bruceman (174), robynmac (177), kr7ysztof (184), mstroz (186), gregepperson (190), roelofse (197), ElinaManninen (198), 101cats (200), RuslanDashinsky (208), OJO_Images (214), MmeEmil (221), Kim_Young (228), monkeybusinessimages (230, 246, 256), RelaxFoto.de (236), bee_photobee (242), Anegada (254), ArtisticCaptures (260), Eskemar (268), og-vision (273), YanLev (278), yaruta (280), Orchidpoet (282), Gorpenyuk (286)
PROOFREADING Eva van Emden

Printed in China

Library and Archives Canada Cataloguing in Publication

Pearson, Liz, 1962-, author
Broccoli, love, and dark chocolate : because food, love, and life should be delicious! / Liz Pearson.

Includes bibliographical references and index.
ISBN 978-1-77050-211-6 (bound)

1. Cooking. 2. Health. 3. Nutrition. 4. Cookbooks. I. Title.

The publisher acknowledges the financial support of the Government of Canada through the Canada Book Fund (CBF) and the Province of British Columbia through the Book Publishing Tax Credit.

14 15 16 17   5 4 3 2 1

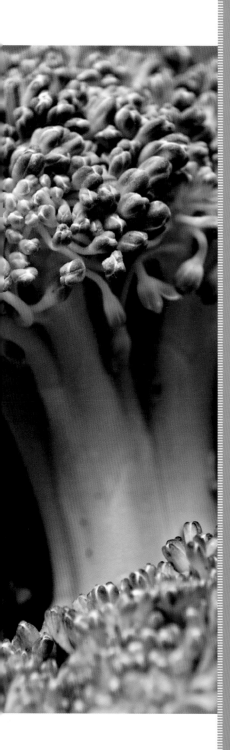

CONTENTS

Acknowledgements

THANKS TO ALL my friends and neighbours who tasted and tested my recipes, including the kids on the street and Teri Boothe.

Thanks to everyone who contributed recipes to this book, including Mairlyn Smith, Amy Snider-Whitson, Sabrina Falone, and Sylvia Kong.

Thanks to Jenny Pearson and Linda Griffiths, who assisted with the food photography.

Thanks to everyone at Whitecap who made this book possible, including Nick Rundall, Jesse Marchand, Theresa Best, Michelle Furbacher, and Jeffrey Bryan.

Thanks to Tracy Bordian who did an exceptional job on the editing and Setareh Ashrafologhalai who did an awesome job on the design.

Last, thanks to my two daughters, Chelsea and Shannon, who supported me, assisted me in the kitchen, and definitely cheered me on.

Get Healthy *and* Happy!

I'VE WRITTEN THREE books and all have received awesome reviews. My last two were national bestsellers and both won awards of excellence (of which I'm very proud). How is this book different? The goal of my last three books was to get you healthy. The goal of this book is to get you healthy *and* happy. How wonderful is that! Life is so much more than just broccoli and dark chocolate. What you eat is important (very important!), but who you are and how you choose to live each day is equally so. I want you and your family to live the best life possible—a life full of laughter, love, good health, and good food. As always, I've included bite-size, reader-friendly, science-backed nutrition information along with totally delicious and easy recipes made with superfood ingredients. The new and exciting part (this is where the happiness part comes in) is the life lessons—you get one with every recipe. The lessons are about love, friendship, gratitude, honesty, courage, and forgiveness, just to name a few. You can learn about food *plus* love and life. Does it get any better? I don't think so!

It's a true honour and privilege to share *Broccoli, Love & Dark Chocolate* with you. May it deliver everything you are looking for and more. Here's to getting a whole lot healthier and a whole lot happier, too!

Sincerely and with love,

LIZ XO

"Because food, love, and life should be delicious!" **LIZ PEARSON, RD**

Top 10 Reasons to Read This Book

1. Your body is the most important home you'll ever live in. Learn how to make it the healthiest and happiest home possible.

2. Superstar foods, such as berries, nuts, and dark leafy greens, can significantly reduce your risk of heart disease, stroke, diabetes, cancer, and dementia, to name a few. Learn how and why to fill your life with superfoods.

3. You can slow down the aging process and even turn back the clock by choosing the right types of foods. Discover which foods are anti-aging all-stars. The quality of your life should be good right up until the end!

4. We are surrounded by food insanity: huge portions, unhealthy ingredients, and a seemingly unlimited availability. Reducing your intake of dietary villains—sugar, sodium, and unhealthy fats—is mandatory for good health. Learn how to minimize your intake of the bad stuff, even on the run.

5. Ever-changing headlines about food and nutrition are frustrating and confusing. One day a food is good for you, the next day, not so good. It's hard to know what to believe. Find solid, science-based answers to your questions. Healthy eating shouldn't be so hard!

6. If you want to look, feel, and be your best, maintaining a healthy body weight matters. Losing weight, however, is tough. Keeping it off is even tougher. Gain insight into weight management and discover strategies that work.

7. Lack of physical activity can kill you, literally! Get educated and inspired to keep your body in motion. If you care about your health, there is no other option.

8. Recipes help put advice into action. The recipes in this book are loaded with all-star, healthy ingredients. Most fit into a busy day. Best of all, each and every recipe passes the "healthy-never-tasted-so-good" test. You'll love them and so will your kids.

9. You should be healthy, but also happy, joyful, and free! That's why each recipe is accompanied by a life lesson. These lessons will inspire you to dream bigger, reach higher, go farther, and let go of all the things in your life that don't serve you well.

10. Everything shared in this book—the advice, the recipes, and the life lessons—comes from a place of love. And many of the life lessons are about love—wonderful, irreplaceable, beautiful love. My hope is that by reading this book, you will love yourself more, love others more, and love your life more, too!

BOTTOM-LINE ADVICE ON — WHAT TO EAT FOR — A LONG AND HEALTHY LIFE

FOODS CAN HARM, foods can heal, and your health matters (a lot!). In Part 1 of this book, my goal is to educate, inspire, and teach you how to choose foods that are all-star protectors of health, including superfoods such as broccoli, kale, almonds, quinoa, blueberries, salmon, dark chocolate, and green tea. You'll understand why minimizing your intake of dietary villains like sugar, salt, and unhealthy fats needs to be a priority. You'll get important questions answered about misunderstood topics such as vitamin supplements, alcohol, gluten-free diets, coffee, organic foods, and probiotics. For people on the go, there's great advice on healthy snacking and dining out. If you want to lose weight and keep it off, you'll learn what works—and what doesn't! This includes important information on staying active. (Did you know sitting is the new smoking?) There's also valuable advice on feeding your family, including children and teens. All of this advice is supported by the latest science and research. This book will help you look good, feel great, and slash your risk of disease. Most importantly, it will help you (and your family!) live a long and healthy life.

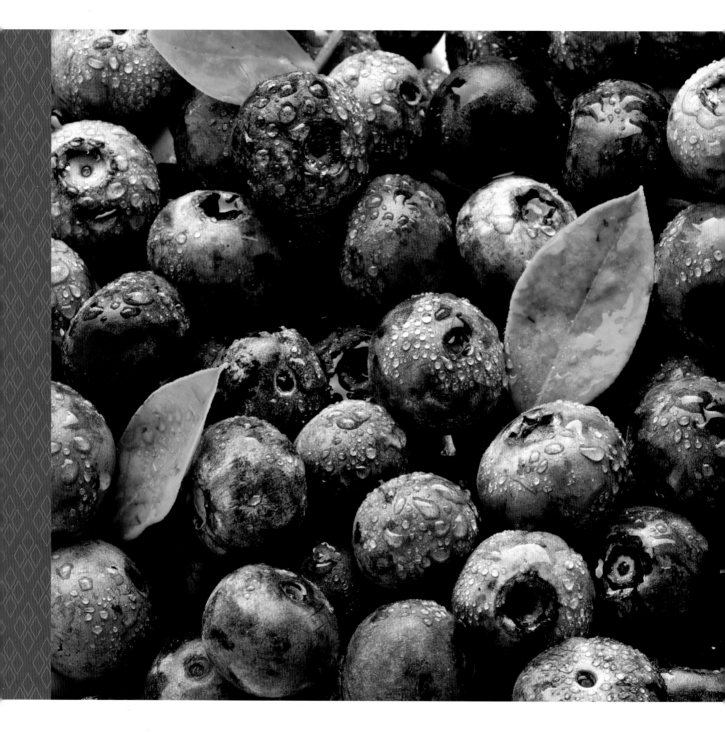

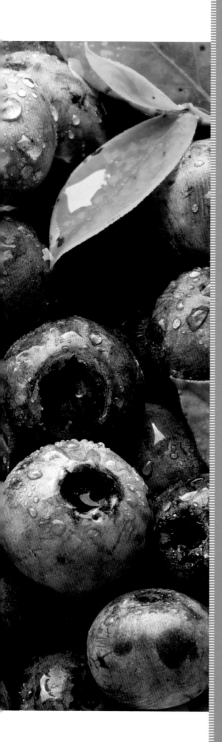

SUPERFOODS

Berries

THE ULTIMATE ANTI-AGING BRAIN FOOD

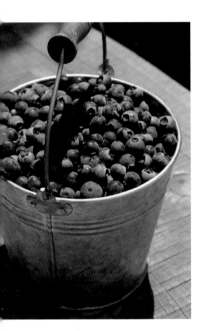

IF YOU LOVE and respect your brain—as well as all of your other body parts—eat berries! They fight inflammation and wage war against harmful free radicals that pummel your body every day. (Free radicals are highly reactive molecules that are produced in the body naturally as a by-product of metabolism and by exposure to toxins such as cigarette smoke and pollution, as well as ultraviolet light. An unhealthy diet and lifestyle also generates free radicals. Antioxidants help neutralize or put free radicals out of business.) Berries protect your brain from damage, as well as your eyes, heart, and skin. In addition to being antioxidant megastars, they're the ultimate anti-aging food: They can slow down the aging process and even turn back the clock. They help to preserve thinking skills and memory, as well as your balance and coordination, as you age. They help defend against cancer, protect your heart, boost immunity, and even help build strong bones.

HELP BRAIN CELLS TALK TO EACH OTHER

By far the best reason to eat berries is to protect your brain. The brain, more than other body parts, is a potential war zone for damage from free radicals. As you get older, this damage can take its toll and affect your ability to think, learn, and remember, and increase your risk of diseases like Alzheimer's. Eating ½ to 1 cup (125 to 250 mL) of berries daily can protect your brain's cells, function, and circuitry, helping to keep your brain young. Berries optimize communication so that when your brain cells talk to each other, the messages get through.

BERRIES KEEP BRAIN CELLS ALIVE

When someone has a stroke, some of their brain cells die. This can result in major disability or even death. Can you protect brain cells from dying? Animal research says yes. Research from the University of South Florida indicates that when berries are included in the daily diet and a stroke is induced, there is a 50% decrease in brain cell death. That's remarkable! Have you had your berries today?

HOUSEKEEPERS FOR THE BRAIN

Have you ever hired someone to clean your house? Eating berries is like hiring someone to clean your brain. Based on a study from the Agricultural Research Service Human Nutrition Research Center on Aging, berries are our brain's natural housekeeper: When you eat them, they activate a mechanism that cleans up a type of toxic debris that can cause memory loss and other mental declines that come with age. If you want a clean brain and a sharp memory, eat your berries!

YOUR BRAIN LIKES BLUE

Research from the University of Manchester says that the majority of debilitating disease is caused in part by poorly bound iron in the body that causes the production of a specific type of harmful, cell-damaging free radical. The good news is that purple or blue fruits like blueberries can't be beat for their ability to bind this iron and prevent it from wreaking havoc on your health. Go, berries, go!

EAT ANTIOXIDANTS AT EVERY MEAL

No matter how pleasant a meal is, eating causes what's known as "oxidative stress"—as we digest our food, we create free radicals that can damage our cells and lead to disease. A study from the Agricultural Research Service in California says eating antioxidant-rich fruits and vegetables, such as berries and dark leafy greens, with each meal helps provide the natural protection against free radicals that our bodies need.

BERRIES SLASH RISK OF HEART ATTACK

Research from Harvard University involving over 93,000 women followed for 18 years found that those who consumed berries three times a week slashed their risk of having a heart attack by one-third. This relationship even held true in women who ate a diet rich in other fruits and vegetables. Your heart loves berries, too!

BERRIES BOOST IMMUNITY

Researchers from the Linus Pauling Institute at Oregon State University analyzed the ability of 446 different compounds to boost the innate or natural immune system in humans. Two compounds stood out from the crowd: pterostilbene (found in blueberries) and resveratrol (found in red grapes). The bottom line: Early research says that if you want to keep your immune system in high gear, make blueberries and grapes a regular part of your eating plan.

CRANBERRIES AND URINARY TRACT INFECTIONS

Cranberries—including cranberry juice, dried cranberries, and even cranberry sauce—help prevent urinary tract infections by stopping bacteria from adhering to the bladder wall. They help prevent stomach ulcers and gum disease the same way. The downside of cranberries is the added sugar they contain. Choose cranberry products with less added sugar when you can.

FOOD *for* THOUGHT
"Blueberries rank among the highest for antioxidant activity in testings of over 100 different foods. Being one of the best sources of antioxidants, blueberries can help slow the aging process and reduce cell damage that can lead to cancer, cardiovascular disease, and loss of brain function."
BRITISH COLUMBIA BLUEBERRY COUNCIL

BERRIES FIGHT CANCER

Carcinogens (cancer-inducing chemicals or substances) can alter our genes and our DNA, causing healthy cells to become unhealthy and replicate. Can berries stop this? In animal research from Ohio State University, a cancer-causing substance altered the activity of some 2,200 genes in only one week, but 460 of those genes were restored to normal when the animals were fed black raspberries as part of their diet during the exposure. What does this tell us? Although one food is probably not enough to prevent cancer—it is the combination of a wide variety of healthy foods that best protect our health—berries should definitely play a prominent part in the mix.

WHICH BERRY IS BEST?

Cornell researchers put wild blueberries at the top of the antioxidant all-stars list. All berries, however, are superheroes for your health. No matter what kind you eat, your body screams "THANK YOU!"

GET MORE BERRIES IN YOUR EATING PLAN

Aim for at least 1 cup (250 mL) of berries daily. Fresh, frozen and dried are all rich sources of antioxidants, but limit your intake of dried berries to ¼ cup (60 mL) a day, as they are more concentrated in sugar and calories. To get more berries in your eating plan, top your cereal with them, mix them into yogurt, or whip them into smoothies. Enjoy them in fruit salads or leafy green salads. Add them to muffins or pancakes. Have them for dessert. Try Strawberries with Balsamic Vinegar, Basil, and Lemon Zest (page 279) and Oatmeal Berry Crisp with Lemon and Maple (page 285). Wild Blueberry Muffins (page 135) and Wild Blueberry Pancakes (page 145) are delicious, too!

ARE EXOTIC BERRIES WORTH THE MONEY?

Are exotic berries such as goji berries (also known as wolfberries) better for you than traditional berries like blueberries? Researchers from Ohio State University compared the cancer-fighting properties of both common berries (blueberries, strawberries, and raspberries) against four other types of more exotic berries (goji, noni, açaí, and black raspberries). Turns out that all berries are about equally effective in helping to prevent cancer. Exotic berries tend to be more expensive and less widely available. The bottom line: Eat a wide variety of berries. Common, traditional berries are always a great choice.

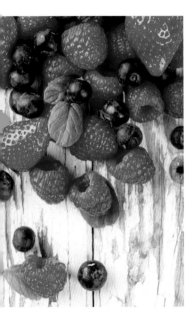

FOOD *for* THOUGHT

"Bioactive compounds from berries have potent antioxidant, anticancer, antimutagenic, antimicrobial, anti-inflammatory, and antineurodegenerative properties."

S. NILE, Konkuk University

LESSON LEARNED

Berries are antioxidant superstars and powerhouse protectors of health, especially brain health. Eat at least 1 cup (250 mL) of berries every day.

An Apple a Day Really Does Keep the Doctor Away

APPLES ARE INEXPENSIVE, portable, and tasty. Best of all, eating just one apple every day provides incredible health protection. What's so special about apples? They're rich in fibre, fill you up, and satisfy hunger better than most other foods. Even more exciting, apples—and especially apple skins—are loaded (and I mean *loaded*) with powerful disease-fighting antioxidant plant compounds called polyphenols, including an especially potent type called procyanidins. Eating apples regularly has been linked to a lower risk of heart disease, stroke, high blood pressure, and cancer. They also protect the aging brain and may reduce the risk of asthma and allergies. Have you eaten an apple today?

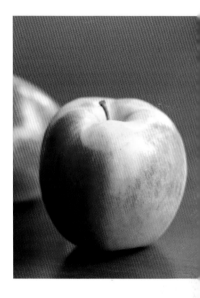

APPLES AND YOUR HEART

Perhaps the best reason to eat apples is to protect your heart. In a study from Ohio State University, healthy middle-aged adults who consumed one apple daily for four weeks significantly lowered blood levels of oxidized LDL (bad) cholesterol.

When LDL cholesterol interacts with free radicals and is oxidized, it becomes especially dangerous. It is more likely to promote inflammation, damage blood vessel walls, and result in hardening of the arteries. Researchers described the study results as "tremendous," stating that daily apple consumption was more effective than other antioxidants they have studied, including those found in turmeric and green tea.

In another study from Florida State University involving 160 women aged 45 to 65, eating two large apples daily for one year lowered LDL (bad) cholesterol by 23% and increased HDL (good) cholesterol by 4%—that's significant! In addition, apple eaters lost on average 3.3 pounds (1.5 kg) of body weight. Other studies also link apples to a lower risk of abdominal or belly fat.

Lastly, in a study from the University of Oxford, researchers concluded that prescribing an apple a day to everyone over 50 could be as effective in reducing the risk of death from heart disease as prescribing a statin (a drug used to lower blood cholesterol).

STRONG CANCER PROTECTION

The plant compounds in apples demonstrate strong cancer-fighting properties. Based on animal research from Cornell

University, eating just one apple a day may considerably lower breast cancer risk in women. Eating two to three apples a day lowers the risk even more. Regular apple eating is also linked to a lower risk of colon, prostate, lung, liver, and skin cancer.

APPLES ARE GOOD FOR YOUR GUT

Animal research from the University of Denmark says apples are very good for gut health. They act as prebiotics and promote the growth of "good" or friendly bacteria along your digestive tract. A healthy gut plays a powerful role in overall health and disease prevention.

PREGNANT WOMEN SHOULD EAT APPLES

Based on research from Utrecht University in the Netherlands involving over 1,200 mothers and their children, women who ate apples during pregnancy reduced the risk of asthma or allergies in their children. Because apples are more likely to contain pesticide residues than most other fruits, eating organic apples, especially during pregnancy, is a wise choice.

APPLES ARE MORE SATISFYING THAN APPLESAUCE OR APPLE JUICE

Research from Pennsylvania State University compared the satiety or fullness factor of apples consumed in different forms. People who ate a whole apple before lunch consumed 15% fewer calories at lunch than those who had applesauce or apple juice. Eating whole apples, including the skin, also offers the best protection for your health by far. Red Delicious and Granny Smith apples are especially high in antioxidants.

GET MORE APPLES IN YOUR EATING PLAN

For something different, try dusting apple slices with cinnamon or serve them with thin slices of reduced-fat aged cheddar cheese. Apple and peanut or almond butter is also a good combo. Try the Apple Pie Muffins (page 133), the Quinoa Salad with Black Beans, Apples, and Red Grapes (page 169), and the Roasted Sweet Potatoes with Apples, Raisins, and Red Onion (page 181). Don't forget to pack an apple every time you head out the door, too!

LESSON LEARNED

Eating one apple every day, with the skin on, is good for your waistline and offers powerful health protection, including a lower risk of heart disease and cancer.

When in Doubt Eat Broccoli
and Leave Some Room for Kale

MY FIRST BOOK was called *When in Doubt, Eat Broccoli! (But leave Some Room for Chocolate)*. Why? Because broccoli is a superstar vegetable! You can't go wrong when you eat it! Broccoli belongs to the cruciferous or brassica family of vegetables. Other vegetables in this group include arugula, bok choy, Brussels sprouts, cabbage, cauliflower, collard greens, horseradish, kale, kohlrabi, mustard greens, radish, rutabaga, turnip, and watercress. Why should you eat them? For their outstanding nutritional value. Broccoli and Brussels sprouts, along with dark leafy greens like kale, are especially high in nutrition, including the powerhouse nutrients vitamin A, vitamin C, vitamin K, beta-carotene, folate, lutein, and zeaxanthin. But that's not all. Cruciferous veggies also fight disease like nobody's business. Their number one claim to fame is their ability to reduce the risk of many types of cancer, including colon, lung, prostate, and breast cancer. They contain plant compounds called isothiocyanates, including sulphoraphane, which help detoxify cancer-causing substances in the body before they do damage. They also activate genes that suppress tumour growth and silence genes that promote cancer development. In addition to being potent cancer fighters, cruciferous vegetables protect against stomach ulcers, respiratory diseases, heart disease, stroke, and osteoarthritis.

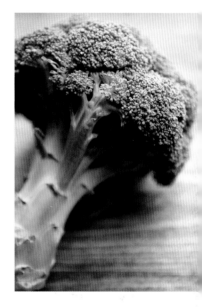

PROTECT YOUR HEART

High blood sugar causes a threefold increase in free radicals that can damage blood vessels and increase the risk of heart disease in people with diabetes. Research from the University of Warwick, however, says the sulphoraphane in broccoli can reduce the formation of free radicals and activate a protein that protects blood vessel walls from damage.

BREATHE EASIER WITH BROCCOLI

UCLA researchers report that broccoli and other cruciferous vegetables can help protect against respiratory inflammation that causes conditions like asthma, allergies, and chronic obstructive pulmonary disease (COPD). The sulforaphane found in these vegetables triggers an increase in antioxidant enzymes in the lungs that offers protection against the onslaught of free radicals in pollution, pollen, and

> **FOOD *for* THOUGHT**
> "Cruciferous vegetables such as broccoli, cauliflower, and cabbage contain a cancer-preventing compound so potent that it is being investigated as a chemotherapy agent."
> **DONALD ABRAMS, MD, Osher Centre for Integrative Medicine**

cigarette smoke that we breathe every day. Free radicals can cause tissue damage, which leads to inflammation and can promote or aggravate these conditions.

BOOST YOUR IMMUNITY

As we get older, our immune system weakens. Want to change that? Eat your broccoli. Based on research from UCLA, compounds in cruciferous vegetables help reduce age-related declines in immune function.

TREATING ARTHRITIS WITH BROCCOLI

Research from the University of East Anglia says that the sulforaphane in broccoli may help prevent or slow down osteoarthritis, the most common form of arthritis. It does this by reducing inflammation and slowing the destruction of cartilage in joints associated with this painful and often debilitating disease.

RAW OR COOKED AND HOW OFTEN?

How many times a week should you eat broccoli and in what form? Most researchers recommend putting broccoli or other cruciferous vegetables, like kale, on the menu at least three to five times a week. Enjoy these vegetables raw or lightly cooked in little or no water. You can steam, microwave, or stir-fry them, but don't boil them—most of the cancer-fighting compounds are water-soluble and will be lost in the water. Cooking broccoli for too long can also destroy

its cancer-fighting power. You should also avoid frozen broccoli. Before freezing, broccoli is blanched, or heated to high temperatures. This inactivates the enzyme that is necessary to form sulforaphane, the powerful cancer-preventive compound in broccoli.

ADD BROCCOLI SPROUTS TO SALADS AND SANDWICHES

Just ½ cup (125 mL) of broccoli sprouts contains as much cancer-fighting sulphoraphane as 6 cups (1.5 L) of broccoli. Wow! Does this mean you should stop eating broccoli? Absolutely not. Broccoli is rich in lots of vitamins, minerals, and fibre not found in sprouts. Best advice: Enjoy both.

BROCCOLI AND DIP

Kids love veggies and dip. They always have and always will. Research from Temple University involving 152 preschool children found that serving broccoli at snack time along with dip increased broccoli consumption by 80% among children who were sensitive to the bitter taste found in some vegetables. That is the power of dip!

GET MORE BROCCOLI AND KALE IN YOUR EATING PLAN

Getting more cruciferous vegetables in your diet has never been so easy or delicious! Two of my favourite ways to enjoy broccoli are grilled on the barbecue (try Grilled Balsamic Broccoli on page 189) or roasted in the oven (try Roasted

FOOD *for* THOUGHT

"While not as well researched as some of its fellow cruciferous vegetables like broccoli or cabbage, kale is a food that you can count on for some unsurpassed health benefits, if for no other reason than its exceptional nutrient richness. Kale is one of the healthiest vegetables around."

THE GEORGE MATELJAN FOUNDATION

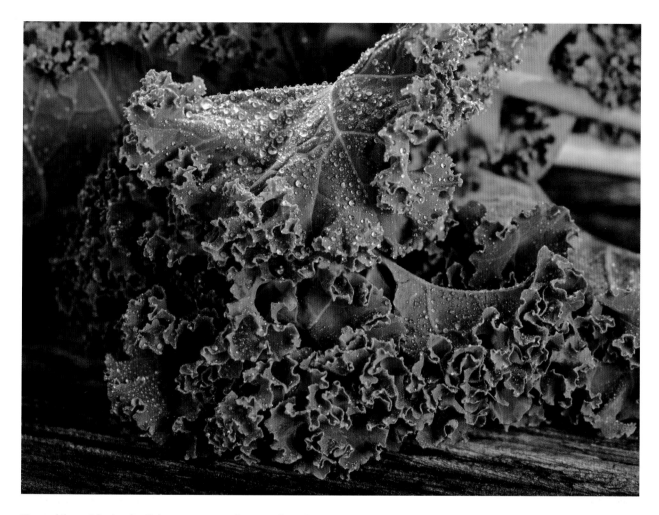

Vegetables with Apple Cider Vinegar and Rosemary on page 173). Relatively new to the market is "baby" kale—it's more tender and sweet than regular kale and is great for salads (see Baby Kale, Cranberry, and Walnut Salad on page 163) and for making roasted kale chips. You can also enjoy kale in a simple sauté with lemon juice, maple syrup, and garlic (page 191) or in a smoothie (page 271).

LESSON LEARNED

Broccoli, kale, and other cruciferous vegetables are nutritional superheroes and disease-fighting superstars, especially when it comes to cancer. Eat them at least three to five times a week.

Dark Leafy Greens Are a Nutritional Goldmine

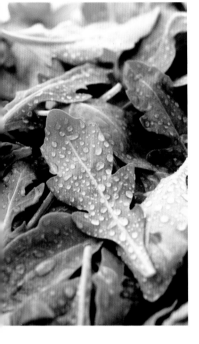

DARK LEAFY GREENS—SUCH as spinach, kale, collard greens, mustard greens, turnip greens, watercress, Swiss chard, and arugula—are often called "green gold" because they contain a goldmine of vitamins, minerals, and valuable plant compounds that fight disease, including magnesium, potassium, vitamin K, vitamin E, folate, and carotenoids (such as beta-carotene, lutein, and zeaxanthin). They are the most nutrient-dense food you can eat, containing more nutrition per calorie than any other food! Eating dark leafy greens regularly can significantly reduce your risk of many diseases, including heart disease and cancer.

GET YOUR VITAMIN K HERE!

It's almost impossible to meet your need for vitamin K if dark leafy greens are not part of your daily diet. Vitamin K is especially important for strong bones and cleaner, healthier arteries. Most multivitamins don't contain it.

PROTECT YOUR EYES WITH GREENS

Vitamin E, lutein, and zeaxanthin—nutrients all found in dark leafy greens—are important for eye health. In a Harvard Nurses' Health Study involving almost 40,000 women, those with the highest intakes of these nutrients were significantly less likely to develop cataracts. Researchers from Ohio State University say these nutrients help protect against sun damage to the eyes that leads to cataracts. Other studies link the nutrients in dark leafy greens to a lower risk of macular degeneration (the leading cause of adult blindness). Bottom line: If you want to see the colour green, eat the colour green!

KEEPING YOUR BRAIN YOUNG

In the Chicago Health and Aging Study, which involved more than 3,700 men and women, those who ate about 3 servings of vegetables daily—green leafy vegetables in particular—had brains that functioned as if they were five years younger. Keep your brain young and eat your greens!

DON'T DRESS YOUR GREENS WITH FAT-FREE DRESSING

Fat helps your body absorb fat-soluble vitamins like A, D, E, and K as well as

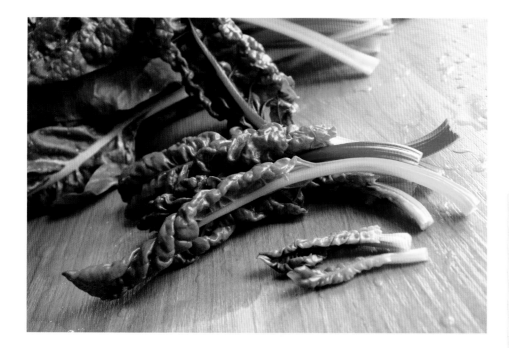

carotenoids such as beta-carotene, lyco-pene, lutein, and zeaxanthin. In a study by Iowa State University, people who ate salad with a fat-free dressing did not absorb any carotenoids, whereas a reduced-fat or full-fat dressing resulted in a substantially greater absorption of these health-protective compounds. The only time a fat-free dressing is okay is when you include other sources of fat (such as nuts, cheese, or avocado) at the same meal or in the salad itself.

LEAFY GREENS AND COUMADIN (WARFARIN)

People who suffer from heart disease often take Coumadin (warfarin), a medi-cation prescribed by their doctor to reduce the risk of blood clots, and are often advised not to eat dark leafy greens because they contain vitamin K, which interferes with this drug. Is this good advice? While it's true that vitamin K helps the blood to clot and can change the way Coumadin works, it doesn't mean you can't enjoy vitamin K-rich foods like dark leafy greens. Simply decide on a consistent quantity of dark leafy greens you're committed to eating daily, get your medication adjusted to complement that amount, and stick to it. Your heart and your health will thank you for it.

DON'T LET GREENS SIT IN THE FRIDGE TOO LONG

The fresher the spinach, the greater the nutritional value. Based on research from Penn State, when spinach is stored in the fridge for eight days, nutrients like folate and beta-carotene can decrease by about 50%. To get the most nutrition from your greens, buy them fresh and

> FOOD *for* THOUGHT
> "I'm strong to the finish when I eats me spinach."
> **POPEYE THE SAILOR MAN**
>
> "Greens are the No. 1 food you can eat regu-larly to help improve your health."
> **JILL NUSSINOW, RD,**
> **Author and Culinary Educator, California**

locally when possible and refrigerate them immediately. Also remember that frozen greens are a great alternative to fresh and are especially great for using in soups and dips.

THE DARKER THE GREEN, THE GREATER THE NUTRITION

How does spinach compare with romaine lettuce? While still a much better choice than iceberg lettuce, romaine pales in comparison to darker greens. Spinach contains twice as much potassium and zinc; three times as much calcium and iron; five times more vitamin K, lutein, and zeaxanthin; six times more magnesium; seven times more vitamin C; and sixteen times more vitamin E. If you are going to go green, why not go dark green?

MICROGREENS OFFER MORE NUTRITION

A new culinary trend is to consume microgreens, the seedlings of dark leafy greens such as spinach and kale. These seedlings are harvested within 14 days of germination when they are only 1 to 3 inches (2.5 to 7.5 cm) in height. They are a wonderful addition to salads, soups, or sandwiches. Researchers from the University of Maryland looked at 25 varieties of microgreens and found that compared with mature leaves, microgreens are even higher in nutritional density.

GET MORE DARK LEAFY GREENS IN YOUR EATING PLAN

If you want to make an investment that pays huge dividends, this is it: Eat at least 1 cup (250 mL) of dark leafy greens each day. Enjoy them in salads, soups, stir-fries, rice, egg, and pasta dishes. Steam them or sauté with extra virgin olive oil, garlic, and herbs. Blend them fresh or frozen into smoothies and dips. Be sure to try Spinach Salad with Blueberries and Almonds (page 161), Rotini Pasta Salad with Honey Ginger Mixed Greens (page 199), and Popeye's Favourite Smoothie (page 269).

LESSON LEARNED

Dark leafy greens are nutritional superstars containing more nutrition per calorie than any other food. You need them for heart health, eye health, brain health, and cancer prevention. Eat at least 1 cup (250 mL) each and every day.

When You Spice Up Your Life, You Spice Up Your Health

HERBS AND SPICES are amazing! Since ancient times they've been used to treat and prevent almost every disease you can name, including heart disease, cancer, and dementia. Considered essential to living a long and healthy life, herbs and spices are antioxidant all-stars. Their ability to prevent harmful, disease-promoting inflammation is second to none, and by killing viruses and bacteria, they can boost your immunity big time. Herbs and spices are also virtually calorie-free and are ideal replacements for the sodium in your diet. Food comes alive with the incredible flavours they provide. Didn't I say they were amazing?

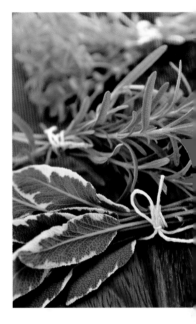

THE SUPER SPICES

All herbs and spices are loaded with health-protective plant compounds that fight disease. The following 12, however, appear to be particularly rich in antioxidants and beneficial plant compounds such as polyphenols. Make every effort to regularly include them in your diet.

Top 12 Super Spices

- allspice
- basil
- cloves
- cinnamon
- ginger
- mint (peppermint, spearmint)
- oregano
- red pepper (including crushed red pepper, cayenne, chili powder, paprika)
- rosemary
- sage
- thyme
- turmeric (found in curry powder)

DON'T FORGET THE ONIONS AND GARLIC

Onions, scallions, leeks, chives, and garlic are all members of the allium family. They are rich in sulfur-containing compounds, as well as flavonoids, and are linked to a lower risk of heart disease and some cancers, especially cancers of the gastrointestinal tract. They also reduce inflammation.

GOOD GARLIC ADVICE

Before you eat, cook, or add garlic to dressings or marinades, be sure to chop or crush it first and then let it sit for 10 minutes. The chopping or crushing activates enzymes that convert garlic compounds into a more health-protective form. Cooking or combining garlic with other ingredients (such as lemon juice) too soon prevents this beneficial activation from taking place.

FOOD *for* THOUGHT

"If you set up a good herb and spice cabinet and season your food liberally, you could double or even triple the medicinal value of your meal without increasing the caloric content."

DIANE HARTLE,
Associate Professor,
University of Georgia

LESSON LEARNED

Herbs, spices, onions, and garlic are loaded with antioxidants and plant compounds that fight disease, reduce inflammation, and boost immunity. They make food more delicious and reduce the need for added salt. Make them a regular part of each and every day.

GOOD ONION ADVICE

Sweeter onions, such as Vidalia, are not as protective for health as regular cooking onions. Onions richer in colour, such as red onions, are higher in antioxidants. Many of the antioxidants are in the outermost layers of onion, so when peeling be sure to remove only the top layers of papery skin. Even a small amount of "overpeeling" can result in the unwanted loss of valuable plant compounds.

ARE FRESH HERBS BETTER THAN DRIED?

Both fresh and dried spices are exceptional sources of antioxidants and provide excellent health benefits. Fresh herbs, however, are more flavourful and generally contain higher levels of antioxidants than dried or processed products. The bottom line: Use fresh when you can, but dried herbs are a convenient and great alternative. When substituting fresh herbs for dried herbs, remember the 3:1 ratio: Use 3 teaspoons (15 mL) of fresh herbs for every 1 teaspoon (5 mL) of dried.

ANTI-INFLAMMATORY ALL-STARS

Chronic inflammation in the body has been linked to a higher risk of most diseases, including heart disease, cancer, dementia, diabetes, and arthritis. Research from the Agricultural Research Service in California suggests that herbs and spices interfere with or block chemical signals or messages sent to and from cells involved in chronic inflammation. Those are some potent anti-inflammatory powers!

5 EASY WAYS TO SPICE IT UP

1. Try the recipes in this book! Most are rich in health-protective spices, onions, and garlic.

2. Grow your own herbs (indoors in winter and outdoors in summer).

3. Buy cookbooks that feature foods from around the world and choose recipes that contain a variety of herbs and spices. Asian, Mediterranean, and Italian cookbooks are a great place to start.

4. Experiment. Start adding more herbs, spices, onions, and garlic to most meals, including salads, salad dressings, vegetable side dishes, and main-course meals.

5. Drink your herbs and spices. Add fresh mint to fruit smoothies. Put cinnamon sticks and sliced ginger in your pot of hot tea. Top lattes or hot chocolate with freshly grated nutmeg.

Nuts

THE EASIEST, MOST CONVENIENT, DELICIOUS SUPERFOOD

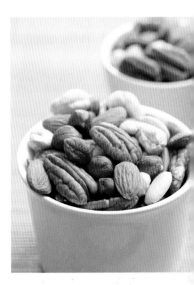

HEALTHY EATING SHOULD be fun, easy, and totally delicious. Which superfood is the most convenient and tastes great, too? Nuts! They're rich in protein and loaded with disease-fighting vitamins, minerals, and fibre, as well as antioxidant-rich plant compounds and heart-healthy fats. They're portable and make the perfect on-the-run snack—no cooking, cleaning, or prep work required. You can also toss them into cereal, salads, rice, vegetable, or pasta dishes. Best of all, they're top-notch protectors of health.

YOUR HEART LOVES NUTS

The research findings on how nuts affect heart health are strong and consistent. Not only do nuts significantly reduce your risk of having a heart attack or stroke, but if you do have one, you're much less likely to die from it. Nuts reduce inflammation and the kind of cholesterol in your blood that clogs your arteries (LDL cholesterol). Nuts also lower your risk of developing type 2 diabetes. If you do suffer from this disease, nuts reduce the risk of diabetes-related complications by helping control blood sugar and blood lipids. Regular nut eaters also have a lower risk of gallstones, cancer, and macular degeneration. Research from the University of Barcelona suggests that eating nuts can even make you feel happier by increasing levels of a feel-good neurotransmitter in the body called serotonin. Nuts truly deserve their superfood status!

YOUR DAILY NUT QUOTA

Nuts are nutritional superstars, but they're also high in calories and fat. Should you be worried? In a review of 33 studies in the *American Journal of Clinical Nutrition*, researchers determined that the regular consumption of nuts is not linked to a higher body weight or a larger waist circumference. This doesn't mean, however, you can eat them all day long. The protein and fibre in nuts is very satisfying—a little goes a long way. Most people (unless you have a very active lifestyle) should limit their intake of nuts to about 1 ounce (30 g) daily. That's about one small handful or ¼ cup (60 mL). If you prefer nut butters, such as peanut or almond butter, keep your daily quota to about 2 tablespoons (30 mL).

FOOD *for* THOUGHT
"In the largest study of its kind, people who ate a daily handful of nuts were 20 percent less likely to die from any cause over a 30-year period than were those who didn't consume nuts."
YING BAO, MD, **Brigham and Women's Hospital**

Here's what 1 serving (1 oz/30 g) of nuts looks like:

- 24 almonds
- 6 to 8 Brazil nuts
- 18 cashews
- 21 hazelnuts
- 10 to 12 macadamia nuts
- 32 peanuts
- 20 pecan halves
- 167 pine nuts
- 47 pistachio nuts
- 14 walnut halves

WHICH NUT IS BEST?

You can't go wrong with almonds or walnuts. Both are backed by lots of great research. Almonds are one of the most nutrient-dense nuts, especially high in magnesium and vitamin E—two powerful, health-protective nutrients most people don't get enough of. Walnuts are chock-full of antioxidants and take top spot for heart-healthy, omega-3 fats. But all nuts offer something special: Brazil nuts lead the pack for cancer-fighting selenium; peanuts are great for folate and protein; hazelnuts contain disease-fighting flavonoids; pecans come loaded with antioxidants and manganese; and pistachios are rich in vitamin B_6. Bottom line: Enjoy a wide variety of nuts, with an emphasis on almonds and walnuts.

A PEANUT BUTTER SANDWICH IS A BEAUTIFUL THING

Peanut butter and other nut butters, such as almond butter, deserve a place in a healthy eating plan. More natural nut butters that don't contain added sugar, salt, or trans fats are a healthier choice, but are not mandatory since the amounts of these added ingredients is generally low. Peanut butter sandwiches are great any time of day, but make a particularly good on-the-run meal when you don't feel like cooking. Be adventurous: Try peanut or almond butter with apple slices, lettuce, raisins, banana, or even kiwi.

MORE HEALTHY NUT-EATING TIPS

- Buy unsalted nuts. You don't need the extra sodium.
- Eat nuts with the skin on (the brown skin on almonds or the papery skin on peanuts, for example). Many health-protective, antioxidant-rich plant compounds are found in the skin.
- Enjoy nuts raw or roasted. Both raw and roasted nuts (whether dry or oil roasted) have similar nutrient contents. Because nuts are already high in healthy fats, they can't absorb much more, even when oil-roasted, so the amount of fat in all types of nuts is similar. Roasting can intensify the flavour and colour, which some people prefer.

WHAT ABOUT SEEDS?

Seeds, including sunflower and pumpkin seeds, offer many of the same health benefits as nuts. Flaxseeds and chia seeds are especially nutritious. They're an excellent source of omega-3 fats and are rich in fibre. Flaxseeds also contain potent plant compounds called lignans, which are linked to a lower risk of heart disease, diabetes, and

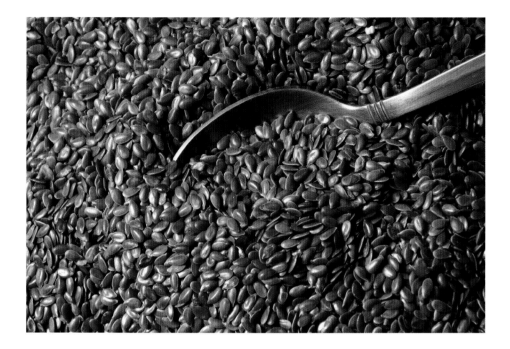

cancer. Eat ground, not whole, flaxseeds for maximum health benefits. Include both nuts and seeds in your daily eating plan. Eat one to two tablespoons (15 to 30 mL) of seeds each day.

FLAXSEEDS LOWER BLOOD PRESSURE

A study by the University of Manitoba involving 110 patients with high blood pressure showed that those who consumed 30 grams (about 4 tablespoons/ 60 mL) of ground flaxseeds every day for six months saw decreases in blood pressure that were the most impressive ever seen in a dietary intervention study. Systolic blood pressure dropped an average 15 mm Hg, and diastolic blood pressure fell an average 8 mm Hg. The bottom line: Flaxseeds lower blood pressure and deliver significant protection against heart attacks and strokes.

LESSON LEARNED

Nuts are the easiest, most convenient superfood you can eat. They're powerful protectors of health, especially heart health. Eat a small handful daily, especially almonds and walnuts. Make seeds, like ground flaxseeds and chia seeds, a regular part of your eating plan too.

Beans

THE BEST HUMAN PLANT FOOD THERE IS

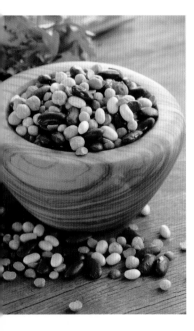

FEW FOODS PROVIDE such an exceptional combination of nutrition, fibre, and health protection as beans (legumes). They deserve a prominent place in any disease-prevention diet. Most people, however, don't eat them as often as they should. Here's why you should make them a priority in your eating plan.

TOP 6 REASONS TO SAY "MORE BEANS, PLEASE!"

1. Bean eaters get more nutrition.
The Nutrient Rich Foods Index developed by the University of Washington ranks food based on nutrient content. Not surprisingly, beans are one of the highest-scoring foods you can eat. Nutritional powerhouses, they are rich in valuable nutrients, including protein, B vitamins, iron, potassium, magnesium, zinc, and copper.

2. Bean eaters get more fibre.
Fibre is a shortfall nutrient, which means the majority of people don't get enough of it. Most of us are getting only about 15 grams of fibre daily when we should be getting 25 grams or more. Just 1 cup (250 mL) of beans contains a whopping 12 to 15 grams of fibre. That's outstanding! Adding beans to your menu makes reaching your daily fibre quota an achievable goal. A high-fibre eating plan has many benefits: It's essential to good gut health, helping to prevent constipation as well as providing important fuel for the "friendly" or good bacteria that live along your gastrointes-tinal tract. Fibre lowers your risk of many diseases, including heart disease, cancer, and diabetes. High-fibre foods fill you up so you eat less food overall.

3. Bean eaters load up on antioxidants that fight disease.
Fruits and vegetables are not the only foods that deserve our attention for their antioxidant status. Beans are also extremely rich in these disease-fighting compounds. Much of their antioxidant activity comes from valuable plant compounds called polyphenols. The key is to go for coloured beans more often—black beans, lentils, pinto beans, and red kidney beans—which contain two to three times more antioxidants than white beans. Antioxidants help stop free radicals from causing damage to body cells that leads to

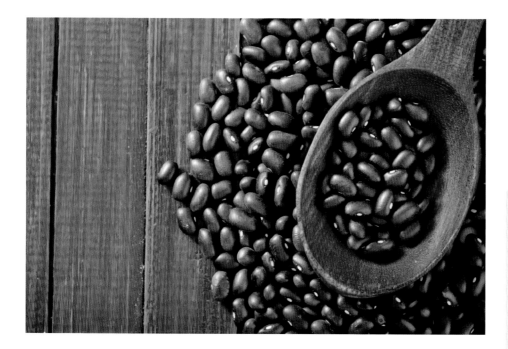

disease, including heart disease, cancer, and dementia.

4. Beans contain slow-release carbs.

Carbohydrates are not the villains! Not if they are "good" carbs. The carbs in beans are about as good as they get. They are released slowly into the bloodstream and provide a long, sustained source of energy. When beans are added to the diets of those who suffer from diabetes, their ability to control their blood sugar is greatly improved. Slowly digested carbs are also linked to significantly lower levels of inflammation in the body. Good carbs are definitely good for overall health!

5. Bean eaters weigh less.

The National Nutrition and Health Examination Survey, a population-wide survey in the United States, reports that people who eat beans four times per week weigh on average about seven pounds less than people who don't eat beans. Regular bean eaters also have less belly fat, the type of fat that is most dangerous to your health. What makes beans so good for your waistline? In addition to helping you feel full longer (due to the protein, fibre, and slow-release carbohydrates they contain), they also appear to affect certain hormones as well as your metabolism, helping you burn calories more efficiently.

6. Bean eaters live longer.

In the Food Habits Later in Life Study, which involved people over the age of 70 in Japan, Sweden, Greece, and Australia, beans were the only food consistently and significantly linked to survival across all populations. It's not surprising when you consider that beans are disease-fighting champions. They are linked to a lower risk of diabetes, some cancers, and especially heart disease. They significantly lower both LDL (bad) cholesterol and blood pressure. More beans, please!

IS SOY HEALTHY?

Soybeans, like all beans, are nutritional superstars. They are unique in that they contain isoflavones, a group of compounds that demonstrate hormone-like activity. While some past research questioned the safety of these compounds, more recent research, including an extensive review by the American Institute of Cancer Research, says that consuming 1 to 2 servings of whole soy foods daily—such as tofu, soy milk, and edamame—definitely fits into a healthy diet and is ultimately linked to a lower risk of disease.

GET MORE BEANS IN YOUR EATING PLAN

With everything beans have going for them, there are simply no excuses for not making every effort to include them in your eating plan at least four times a week. Make a big batch of chili. Enjoy bean salads and bean dips, including hummus. Add beans to rice and pasta dishes. Learn to cook with beans. Try the multitude of bean recipes in this book, including Liz's Award-Winning Chili (page 217), Black Bean, Corn, and Mango Fiesta Salad (page 213), Rosemary Roasted Chickpeas (page 221), Spicy Red Lentil Soup (page 155), and Dried Apricot and Greek Yogurt Hummus (page 257). However you enjoy them, feel good knowing that eating more beans is a wonderful way to take care of yourself.

LESSON LEARNED

Beans are nutritional powerhouses loaded with nutrients, fibre, antioxidants, and slowly digested carbohydrates. Regular bean eaters weigh less, have a significantly lower risk of disease, and live longer. Eat beans at least four times a week.

Whole Grains Protect Health; Refined Grains Harm Health

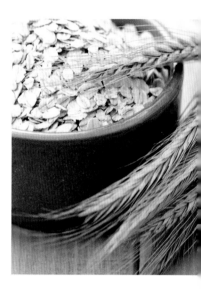

WHOLE GRAINS ARE disease-fighting superstars that contain a complex mix of vitamins, minerals, fibre, and health-protective plant compounds like phenolics and flavonoids. For optimal health, it's essential to eat the "whole" grain. When refined grain products are made—like white bread or white rice—the bran and germ portion of the grain are discarded, and with them much of the health-protective power.

5 GREAT REASONS TO MAKE EVERY DAY A WHOLE-GRAIN DAY

1. Whole grains are highly nutritious and contain antioxidants.

Adults, teens, and children who eat more whole grains have better-quality diets and nutrient intakes. Whole-grain products are significantly higher in many vitamins and minerals than products made with refined grains. For example, compared with white flour, whole-wheat flour contains:

- twice as much calcium and selenium
- three times more copper, phosphorus, potassium, and choline
- four times more zinc and fibre
- six times more magnesium, manganese, and vitamin K
- twelve times more vitamin E, lutein, and zeaxanthin

In addition, more than 80% of the disease-fighting antioxidants are found in the bran or germ fraction of the whole grain (based on research from Cornell University). The antioxidant content of whole grains rivals or exceeds that of fruits and vegetables. Bottom line: With whole grains you get a whole lot more!

2. Whole-grain eaters have less belly fat.

In a study conducted by Pennsylvania State University, 50 obese adults consumed a reduced-calorie diet for 12 weeks. Half the group was asked to eat only whole grains as part of their diet, and the other half was asked to eat only refined grains. The whole-grain eaters saw a significantly greater decrease in abdominal fat as well as a 38% decrease in C-reactive protein, an inflammatory marker for heart disease. This is consistent with a review of 15 studies by London researchers involving almost 120,000 men and women. They found that those who consumed more whole grains (about 3 servings a day) had a lower body weight and less central obesity (belly fat). Whole-grain eaters are also less likely to gain weight as they age.

3. Whole grains are good for gut health.

A whole-grain eating plan is linked to a lower risk of cancer, especially cancers of the gastrointestinal tract such as colon and rectal cancer. Whole grains are an important source of fibre and act as prebiotics in the gut by stimulating the growth of "good" or friendly bacteria that live there and provide strong protection against disease.

4. Whole grains slash your risk of heart attack, stroke, and high blood pressure.

Whole grains reduce heart disease risk by lowering blood pressure and blood cholesterol and reducing plaque buildup on artery walls. In a study from the University of Aberdeen in the UK, eating 3 servings of whole grains a day was linked to decreases in blood pressure as significant as using blood pressure lowering drugs. In another study from Wake Forest University in North Carolina, researchers measured atherosclerosis (plaque buildup) of the common carotid artery (the major artery going to the head and neck), in over 1,100 men and women. Researchers concluded that those who ate more whole grains had less unhealthy thickening of the artery wall.

5. Whole grains are linked to a lower risk of diabetes.

A Harvard University study involving almost 200,000 men and women concluded that eating white rice five or more times a week was linked to an increased risk of type 2 diabetes, while eating brown rice two or more times a week was linked to a lower risk. They estimate that replacing about 2 servings a week of white rice with the same amount of brown rice would lower diabetes risk by 16%.

IS IT A WHOLE GRAIN?

The healthiest diets contain a wide variety of different whole grains, including:

- amaranth
- brown rice and coloured rice (black, purple, red)
- buckwheat
- corn (including whole-grain cornmeal and popcorn)
- hulled barley
- millet
- oats (including oatmeal)
- quinoa
- teff
- whole rye
- whole wheat (including varieties such as spelt, emmer, farro, einkorn, Kamut®, durum and forms such as bulgur or cracked wheat and wheatberries)

- whole-grain sorghum (also called milo)
- whole-grain triticale
- wild rice

DON'T BE FOOLED!
BECOME AN EXPERT WHOLE-GRAIN LABEL READER

Food companies are savvy. They know how to make many foods *look like* they are whole grain even when they are not. Here are some tips to help you navigate the labelling:

- Look for "100% whole grain" on the front of the package. Products that say "made with" whole wheat or another whole grain may contain more refined grains, such as white flour, than whole grains.
- Don't use colour to guide you. Some breads, including many rye and pumpernickel breads, are brown because of molasses or other added ingredients. Make sure all of the grains listed on the ingredient list are whole grains.
- Don't buy products that include wheat flour (or enriched wheat flour or unbleached wheat flour) on the ingredient list. This is another name for white flour. In Canada look for "whole-grain whole-wheat flour" (if it says just whole wheat, part of the germ may have been removed). In the United States "whole-wheat flour" does mean it is 100% whole grain. Rolled, instant, quick, or steel-cut oats all qualify as whole grains.

Degerminated or degermed corn or cornmeal is not a whole grain. Neither is pearled barley.

- Multi-grain, 12-grain, or 7-grain doesn't mean 100% whole grain. White flour could be a primary ingredient. Check the ingredient list and make sure all the grains are whole grains.
- To help people easily identify whole-grain products, the Whole Grains Council developed a whole-grain stamp. Some foods carry it. The stamp tells you how many grams of whole grains the product contains. One stamp says "whole grain: 8 grams or more per serving" (which means the product contains at least a half serving of whole grains) and the other stamp says "100% whole grain: 16 grams or more per serving" (which means the product contains a full serving of whole grains).
- Breads, cereals, and other grains are a major source of sodium in the diet for many people. Compare labels and choose brands that are lower both in sodium and in added sugar.

LESS PROCESSED WHOLE GRAINS ARE BETTER FOR YOU

The common processing of whole grains—which can involve grinding, puffing, and flaking them—can impact their healthfulness, including a loss of some of the natural antioxidants and fibre. This processing can also cause the sugars in the grain to be released into the bloodstream much more quickly, causing a spike or rapid rise in

FOOD *for* THOUGHT
There is consistent epidemiological evidence that whole-grain foods substantially lower the risk of chronic diseases such as cardiovascular disease, diabetes, and cancer and also play a role in body weight management and digestive health.
SUMMARY OF AMERICAN SOCIETY FOR NUTRITION SATELLITE SYMPOSIUM

blood sugar followed by a quick fall. Less processed whole grains, like steel-cut oats, wheatberries, barley, millet, and quinoa, are digested slower and result in a more gradual and healthier rise in blood sugar, which lowers your overall risk of disease and leaves you feeling full longer. In a study from Children's Hospital in Boston, boys who ate instant oatmeal at breakfast had much larger blood sugar spikes and ate 53% more calories at lunch than boys who ate steel-cut oats (a less-processed form of oats). The bottom line: Choose more intact, less processed grains whenever possible.

CHOOSING HEALTHIER BREADS, CEREALS, AND CRACKERS

Want a simple way to choose healthier processed whole-grains products, such as bread, cereals, and crackers? Use the 10:1 ratio as recommended by Harvard researchers: Read product labels and choose products that contain at least 1 gram of fibre for every 10 grams of carbohydrate. For example, if a whole-grain bagel contains 30 grams of carbohydrates, it should contain at least 3 grams of fibre or more.

IS WHITE WHOLE-WHEAT BREAD REALLY GOOD FOR YOU?

Relatively new to the market are breads and other products made with "white" whole wheat rather than the traditional "red" whole wheat used to make most whole-wheat products. White whole wheat has the same amount of fibre, vitamins, and minerals as red whole wheat, but its bran layer is lower in beneficial antioxidant plant compounds. Animal studies from the University of Minnesota suggest that red whole wheat does a better job of reducing the risk of colon cancer. Some people, however, prefer the milder taste of white whole wheat.

THE BENEFITS OF SPROUTED GRAINS

Can the process of soaking and sprouting grains boost their nutritive powers? It appears the answer is yes, although much of the research is still in the early stages. Sprouted grains and products made with sprouted grains, such as bread, may contain more vitamins, minerals, and antioxidants, as well as less gluten. They may be easier to digest and also less likely to cause allergies. Ongoing research will tell us more.

GET MORE WHOLE GRAINS IN YOUR EATING PLAN

Give whole grains a chance. The first time people try whole-grain pasta, for example, they may find the taste is different than what they are used to. After eating it a few times, however, many people prefer the fuller, nuttier taste. Give yourself time to adjust, adapt, and enjoy! Here are some especially delicious whole-grain dishes I'm sure you'll love: Mediterranean-Herbed Brown Rice and Lentil Salad (page 203), Tuscan Supper (page 207), and Totally Terrific Tex-Mex Bow-Tie Pasta (page 195).

LESSON LEARNED

Most people eat enough grains, but fail to choose whole grains. Whole grains offer significantly more nutrition, fibre, and antioxidants than refined grains. This results in significantly greater protection from disease, including heart disease, diabetes, and cancer. Whole-grain eaters are also more likely to maintain a healthy body weight. Choose less processed, intact whole grains most often.

Fibre

OUR ANCESTORS ATE IT
AND WE NEED MORE OF IT

FIBRE IS FOUND in plant foods, and our ancestors' diet was loaded with it. Today's highly processed diets are fibre-deficient. Almost all children, teens, and adults get half as much as they need. You want fibre and lots of it! Here's why: Your body can't digest or absorb it, so it works as both a broom and a sponge as it moves along your digestive tract. It reduces your risk of colon cancer as well as constipation, hemorrhoids, and diverticular disease (small pouches that form in your colon). It lowers LDL (bad) cholesterol and blood pressure, and helps prevent spikes in blood sugar after eating. It keeps your appetite under control by making you feel full longer. It is definitely good for health!

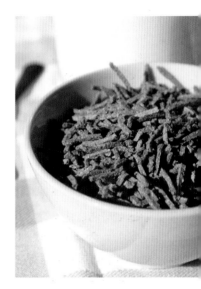

LOWER YOUR LIFETIME
RISK OF HEART DISEASE

If you want to avoid heart disease later in life, load up on fibre now—that's the result of a study done by Northwestern Medicine involving about 11,000 men and women. Those who had the highest fibre intake had a significantly lower lifetime risk of heart disease compared with those who had the lowest fibre intake.

FIBRE BLASTS BELLY FAT

According to research from Wake Forest Baptist Medical Center, if you want to get rid of abdominal or belly fat—the type of fat that's most dangerous to your health— eat more soluble fibre. Good sources of soluble fibre include oats, barley, rye, psyllium, flaxseeds, beans, apples, pears, and citrus fruits. Soluble fibre, which is best known for lowering blood cholesterol and blood sugar levels, has also been linked to a healthier immune system, including a faster recovery from infection.

MORE FIBRE MEANS
LESS WEIGHT GAIN

In a Harvard Nurses' Health Study involving about 75,000 women, those who had the highest fibre intake were almost 50% less likely to experience major weight gain over a 12-year period. Researchers estimated that women who increased their fibre intake by 12 grams (to reach a total of about 25 grams) gained about 8 pounds (3.5 kg) less than women with lower fibre intakes.

SLASH YOUR RISK OF STROKE

Want to protect your brain and slash your

LESSON LEARNED

Fibre is a health-protecting nutrient few people get enough of. It's especially important for digestive and heart health, as well as appetite and blood sugar control. High-fibre bran cereals and beans are exceptionally rich sources, but fruits, vegetables, whole grains, nuts, and seeds are also good choices.

risk of stroke? Researchers from the University of Leeds reviewed eight studies and concluded that every 7-gram increase in daily fibre intake reduces the risk of a first stroke by 7%. As fibre intake goes up, stroke risk goes down.

YOUR GUT LOVES FIBRE!

A study from the University of Illinois shows that eating more fibre and different types of fibre encourages more beneficial bacteria to flourish in your gut. These "good" bacteria support a healthy gastrointestinal tract and may reduce the risk of a long list of diseases, including colon cancer, inflammatory bowel disease, type 2 diabetes, and rheumatoid arthritis.

WHAT'S YOUR MINIMUM DAILY FIBRE QUOTA?

- Children ages 1 to 8   19 to 25 grams
- Females ages 9 to 50   25 grams
- Females over 50   21 grams
- Males ages 9 to 50   31 to 38 grams
- Males over 50   21 grams

THE BEST WAY TO MEET YOUR FIBRE QUOTA

- High-fibre bran cereals (such as All-Bran, Bran Buds, Fiber One, and Fibre First) can't be beat. They contain a whopping 12 to 18 grams of fibre per ½ cup (125 mL) serving. Wow!
- Beans or legumes are high-fibre superstars, containing as much as 15 grams of fibre per 1 cup (250 mL). Another wow!

- Load up on fruits and vegetables and always eat them with the skin on. Some especially good choices include apples, berries (especially raspberries and blackberries), dried fruits (apricots, dates, figs, prunes, raisins), pears, artichokes, and peas.
- Make nuts and seeds a regular part of your day, including ground flaxseeds and chia seeds.
- Swap all the refined grains (such as white bread) in your diet with whole grains. Hulled barley, bulgur, and wheat berries are especially high in fibre.
- Read labels and choose high-fibre foods more often. Choose products that contain a minimum of 2 to 3 grams of fibre per serving and ideally 4 to 6 grams of fibre or more.

GRADUALLY INCREASE YOUR INTAKE

If your current eating plan is lacking in fibre, don't add too much too quickly as it could lead to bloating, cramping, or gas. Add it gradually over a few weeks and drink lots of water. Fibre absorbs water and does its best work when accompanied by plenty of it.

Olive Oil Is Exceptional

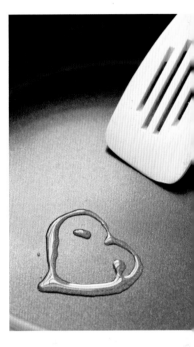

"FAT" USED TO be a nasty word in the world of food. Not any more. We now know there are goods fats that can protect health and bad fats that can harm health. Polyunsaturated and monounsaturated fats found in many vegetable oils, higher-fat fish, nuts, and avocados fall into the good fat category. Saturated fats found in higher-fat milk products and fatty meats are not so good. Trans fats found in some processed and deep-fried foods are terrible. The omega-3 fats from fish are all-star health protectors (see page 35). Where does extra virgin olive oil fit in? It is an exceptionally good fat. It fights disease, saves lives, and can help you lead a longer, healthier life.

EXTRA VIRGIN OLIVE OIL IS #1

In terms of which of the added fats—the fats you use in cooking, salad dressings, and marinades, for example—are good for you, extra virgin olive oil wins by a huge margin. Significantly more research supports the use of extra virgin olive oil over any other oil.

Extra virgin olive oil is:

- rich in monounsaturated fat, a healthy fat
- loaded with plant compounds called phenols that demonstrate potent antioxidant, anti-microbial, and anti-inflammatory properties
- an integral part of the traditional Mediterranean diet, which is proven to protect health and promote longevity and is linked to a significantly lower risk of many diseases, including heart disease, cancer, and Alzheimer's disease

Canola oil, my second choice or back-up oil, is:

- rich in monounsaturated fat and one of the best plant sources of omega-3 fats
- lower in saturated fat than most oils
- has a relatively balanced ratio of omega-3 to omega-6 fats

OLIVE OIL AND YOUR GUT

Recent studies have linked extra virgin olive oil to a lower risk of digestive disorders, including inflammatory bowel disease. In research done by the University of East Anglia in the UK involving more than 25,000 people, those with the highest intakes of olive oil (about 2 to 3 tablespoons/30 to 45 mL daily) had a 90% lower risk of developing ulcerative colitis. Olive oil appears to block chemicals in the bowel that aggravate inflammation.

OLIVE OIL FOR A HEALTHY BRAIN

Several studies link the Mediterranean diet to a lower risk of dementia. Extra virgin olive oil appears to protect cells in the brain from the normal deterioration associated with aging, as well as guard against the type of damage that leads to Alzheimer's disease. It helps decrease the accumulation of beta-amyloid in the brain, which is a key culprit in the development of Alzheimer's.

YOUR HEART LOVES OLIVE OIL

At the end of the 1950s, the Seven Countries Study looked at rates of heart disease and eating habits around the world. The results were fascinating. Both the United States and the island of Crete in the Mediterranean were getting about 40% of their calories from fat. The rates of heart disease for the American men, however, was more than 30 times higher than for the men living in Crete. The fat in the American diet was primarily saturated fat that came from meat and high-fat dairy, while the fat in the Mediterranean diet came primarily from extra virgin olive oil. Bottom line: It is the type of fat, not the quantity, that has the greatest impact on health.

OLIVE OIL SLASHES STROKE RISK

In the Three City Study from France involving almost 9,000 people age 65 and older followed for more than five years, those who consumed the most extra virgin olive oil (used for cooking, in salad dressings, and as a dip for bread) reduced their risk of stroke by more than 70% compared with those who didn't use olive oil.

MAKE IT "EXTRA VIRGIN" OLIVE OIL

In the EurOlive study, researchers recruited 200 healthy men and randomly assigned them to one of three groups to consume 1 tablespoon (15 mL) of olive oil containing low, medium, or high amounts of phenols every day for three weeks. (Phenols are the health-protective antioxidant plant compounds found in higher amounts in extra virgin olive oil.) The results showed that as the level of phenols increased, the amount of oxidized LDL (bad) cholesterol in the blood decreased. When LDL becomes oxidized or damaged it is much more likely to cause plaque to build up on the artery wall. Other studies have also found that as the phenol content of olive oil increases, so does its ability to reduce inflammation and to increase your HDL (good) cholesterol, the kind that helps carry cholesterol out of your bloodstream and to your liver for disposal. Bottom line: For cleaner arteries, don't use any kind of olive oil, use "extra virgin" olive oil.

FOOD *for* THOUGHT
"Olive oil is a hotter commodity than ever thanks to research linking it to good health and wellness. Many nutrition experts recommend that your first choice in oils—for cooking or cold preparations—be extra virgin olive oil."
SHARON PALMNER, RD,
Columnist, *Today's*
Dietitian

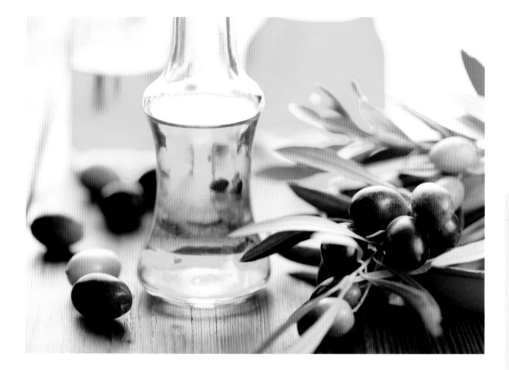

FIGHT THE FIRE WITH OLIVE OIL

Chronic inflammation in the body is linked to a higher risk of heart disease, cancer, diabetes, arthritis, and Alzheimer's disease. The phenols in extra virgin olive oil have potent anti-inflammatory properties. A study by the University of Cordoba in Spain revealed that a diet high in phenol-rich olive oil changed the way 98 different genes functioned in the body. That's amazing! Olive oil was able to turn off some of the genes that promote inflammation. Three cheers for extra virgin olive oil!

CANCER PREVENTION WITH OLIVE OIL

Researchers from Milan, Italy, reviewed 25 studies on olive oil consumption and cancer risk. Olive oil was linked to a significantly lower risk of cancers of the breast, respiratory tract, and upper digestive tract. In fact, the risk of cancer was as much as five times lower in people who consumed mainly olive oil compared with those who consumed mainly butter. A different review by the University of Athens looked at 38 studies involving over 37,000 people and found that those who consumed the most olive oil had a 34% lower risk of developing any type of cancer. Olive oil prevents cell damage by free radicals that leads to cancer, inhibits cancer cell growth, and promotes cancer cell death. Didn't I say it was a good fat?

OLIVE OIL FOR STRONG BONES

The olive oil consumed as part of the Mediterranean diet is linked to healthier bones. Researchers from Spain report that

FOOD *for* THOUGHT

"Olive oil is an integral ingredient in the Mediterranean diet. There is growing evidence that it may have great health benefits including the reduction in coronary heart disease risk, the prevention of some cancers, and the modification of immune and inflammatory responses."

MOHAMED HAMMAMI, Researcher, University of Monastir

olive oil increases blood levels of osteocalcin, which is a calcium-binding protein important for strong bones.

THE TASTE OF LIQUID GOLD

Why be a wine connoisseur when you can be an olive oil connoisseur? Many gourmet food shops invite you to sample olive oils. Take the time to taste the incredible variety of flavours. Like wine, the flavour of olive oil, especially extra virgin olive oil, is affected by many factors, including the type and ripeness of the olive and the growing conditions. When cooking or stir-frying with olive oil, use a medium heat, not a high heat, to help preserve its wonderful flavour.

MORE ANTIOXIDANTS, PLEASE!

Buy only extra virgin olive oil. It is much higher in health-protective antioxidants. The fresher the olive oil, the better. Look for brands that indicate the date it was packaged. According to a study from Italy, the potency of antioxidants can decline as much as 40% after six months of sitting on the shelf. Olive oil is sensitive to heat and light, so store it in a cool, dark cupboard.

HOW MUCH SHOULD YOU CONSUME?

Based on the Mediterranean diet and current research, you should consume about 1 to 2 tablespoons (15 to 30 mL) of extra virgin olive oil a day. Dip your bread into it. Use it in salad dressings and marinades and when you stir-fry or sauté.

WHAT ABOUT COCONUT OIL?

Coconut oil is high in saturated fat. The type of saturated fat found in coconut oil (primarily lauric acid) does not appear to be as detrimental to health as the kind found in milk products, meat, and palm oil. The degree to which coconut oil may actually protect health, however, is another question. There is currently a lack of good, solid research in this area. If you use coconut oil, use it in small quantities. Far more research says most of your fats should come from extra virgin olive oil, nuts, seeds, and fatty fish.

LESSON LEARNED

Extra virgin olive oil is rich in healthy fats and loaded with valuable plant compounds that significantly lower your risk of disease, including heart disease, cancer, and dementia. Make it the primary source of added fat in your diet.

Fish May Be the Most Important Food You Can Eat for Your Health

OMEGA-3 FATS FROM higher-fat fish—salmon, rainbow trout, mackerel, herring, and sardines—change the composition of our bodies. These fats get incorporated into all of our cell membranes, including our heart, blood vessels, eyes, and brain, and work their magic, protecting our cells from damage and reducing the kind of inflammation that leads to disease. They totally transform the way our cells react, respond, and communicate with each other. Omega-3 fats are linked to a lower risk of many diseases and disorders, including heart disease, stroke, Alzheimer's, cancer, depression, arthritis, asthma, allergies, and macular degeneration. They are an absolute must-have in any diet designed for a long and healthy life.

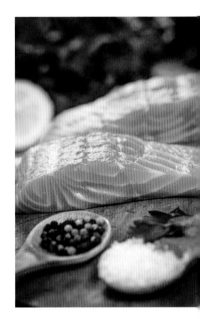

OMEGA-3 FATS FROM PLANTS ARE NOT THE SAME

Plant foods like walnuts, canola oil, and flaxseeds contain an omega-3 fat called alpha-linolenic acid (ALA). The omega-3 fats found in fish or seafood are called eicosapentaenoic acid (EPA) and docosahexaenoic acid (DHA). Although all types of omega-3 fats are beneficial for health, the plant source omega-3 fats are not linked to nearly as many health benefits. They don't get incorporated into cell membranes the same way that marine or fish source omega-3 fats do. For optimal health, both plant source and marine source omega-3 fats are a must!

RESEARCHER DISCOVERS THE POWER OF FISH

In the 1970s researchers wanted to know why the Greenland Inuit had one of the lowest rates of death from heart disease on the planet—only about 5% of their adult male population was dying from heart disease compared with 40% in the United States. The answer: Their diet was loaded with fish and seal meat and, therefore, omega-3 fats. No other food protects the heart and blood vessels like the omega-3 fats from fish. Not only are you much less likely to suffer from a heart attack or stroke, but if you do, these fats help protect the heart and brain from damage and play an important role in the recovery process.

FOOD *for* THOUGHT

"Fish, such as salmon, are as potentially potent as any high-tech heart drug."

ALEXANDER LEAF, MD, **Harvard Medical School**

OMEGA-3 FATS PROMOTE PLAQUE STABILITY

Unstable plaque is more likely to rupture, leading to a heart attack or stroke. Researchers from the University of Southampton in the UK took 162 patients waiting to have surgery to remove plaque from their carotid artery (the main artery leading from the heart to the brain) and, for an average of 42 days prior to the surgery, gave part of the group daily fish oil capsules. The result: The patients who took the fish oil had fewer plaques with thin fibrous caps and signs of inflammation and more plaques with thick fibrous caps and no signs of inflammation. Bottom line: For more stable plaque, eat fish.

FISH FIGHTS CANCER

Animal research at the University of Guelph indicates that a lifelong diet rich in omega-3 fats from fish can significantly reduce the risk of breast cancer. This study is said to provide unequivocal evidence that omega-3s reduce cancer risk. Researchers found that omega-3 fats cut the risk of cancer development by one-third and tumours that did form were about 30% smaller.

FISH OIL FOR ARTHRITIS

More than a dozen studies have found that high doses of fish oil supplements taken long term and with pain medication can reduce joint swelling, ease

morning stiffness, and lessen fatigue in people with rheumatoid arthritis. Fish oil has been shown to help people with osteo-arthritis, too.

AGE SLOWER

Want to protect your cells from aging? Eat fish. At the ends of our DNA (the blueprint our cells use to reproduce) there are protective caps called "telomeres." Longer telomeres are linked to younger cells and a longer life. In a five-year study conducted by the University of California, patients with heart disease who had higher blood levels of omega-3 fats experienced a much slower shortening of telomere length, while those with the lowest blood levels of omega-3 fats experienced a rapid rate of telomere shortening. In other words, the cells of people with higher intakes of omega-3 fats seemed to age at a much slower rate.

FISH REALLY IS BRAIN FOOD

About 60% of the human brain is made up of fat. Healthy fats, especially the omega-3 fats from fish, make for a healthier brain. A brain cell that is high in these omega-3 fats is virtually liquid and has more branches, allowing for more effective reception and communication. Regular consumption of omega-3 fats from fish is linked to better brain development during childhood, a lower risk of depression throughout life, and the maintenance of cognitive function later in life (the ability to think and learn), including a lower risk

FOOD *for* THOUGHT

"Every so often, scientists really do discover a substance of transformative power, one with the ability to cure the previously incurable and improve the quality of life for the rest of us. Omega-3 fatty acids—a component of simple fish oil once so prevalent in our diet but now largely absent—could be such a substance."

ANDREW STOLL, MD,
Harvard Medical School

of dementia and Alzheimer's disease.

PREGNANT WOMEN NEED FISH

Pregnant women who regularly consume omega-3 fats from fish are less likely to suffer from postpartum depression, have fewer premature births, and have babies with healthier birth weights. These fats are critical to the developing brain, nerve, and eye cells of the child and can affect a child's ability to think, learn, and focus throughout life. Some pregnant women avoid fish for fear of contaminants. The best decision is to choose the safest fish to eat (see page 39) or take fish oil capsules, as studies show they are low in contaminants. Omega-3 fats from fish are essential for the health of both mother and child.

"HAPPY FATS"

The omega-3 fats from fish impact neurochemical pathways in the brain that affect mood, including the release of serotonin, a mood regulator. A review of 15 studies by the New York State Psychiatric Institute concluded that the omega-3 fats from fish reduce the risk of depression. Another review of five studies by the University of Melbourne concluded these fats help treat bipolar depression. When researchers looked at 23 countries around the world, they found that new moms who ate more fish were less likely to suffer postpartum blues. Omega-3 fats have also been linked to a lower risk of aggression, impulsivity, and attention-deficit/hyperactivity

disorder (ADHD). Bottom line: Don't worry, be happy—eat fish!

SEAFOOD HELPS YOU SEE

High concentrations of omega-3 fats are found in the eye's retina and are essential to eye health. In a 10-year Harvard study involving almost 40,000 women, those who consumed 1 or more servings of fish per week (especially higher-fat fish) were 42% less likely to develop age-related macular degeneration, the leading cause of adult blindness.

PROTECT YOUR HEARING WITH FISH

Hearing loss is a significant burden that often comes with age. Could eating fish make a difference? Early research says yes. In the Blue Mountains Hearing Study, which involved almost 3,000 participants aged 50 and older, eating 1 to 2 servings of fish a week was linked to a 42% lower risk of hearing loss. Omega-3 fats are thought to protect hearing by promoting good blood flow to the inner ear.

BOOST YOUR IMMUNITY WITH FISH

Want to get sick less often? Eat fish. Based on animal research from Michigan State University, fish oil boosts immunity by enhancing B cell activation and antibody production, which helps clear bacteria or viruses from your body. Is there anything fish oil doesn't do? I don't think so!

FOOD *for* THOUGHT
"Seafood is likely the single most important food one can consume for good health."
DARIUSH MOZAFFARIAN, Professor, Harvard School of Public Health

SHOULD YOU BUY SUPPLEMENTS THAT CONTAIN OMEGA 3-6-9 FATS?

No. Most people get more than enough omega-6 and omega-9 fats through diet. Getting too much omega-6 fats can also diminish the benefits you get from omega-3 fats. Stick to the omega-3 fats that come from fish oil. It is the nutrient that most people don't get nearly enough of.

FISH OIL ON TRIAL

The GISSI trial is one of the largest population studies to look at the benefits of taking fish oil capsules to combat the risk of heart disease. In this study involving over 11,000 Italian men and women with pre-existing heart disease, those who took 1 gram of fish oil every day slashed their risk of dying from a heart attack by 45%.

HOW MUCH FISH AND/OR FISH OIL SHOULD YOU CONSUME?

- Aim for 2 servings of higher-fat fish (such as salmon, trout, mackerel, herring, or sardines) each week. Anchovies and pickled herring are high in omega-3 fats, but are also high in sodium, so be wary. In addition to omega-3 fats, fish is a protein-rich, nutrient-rich food.
- One serving of fish is equal to: 3 to 4 ounces (85 to 110 g) of fish—about the size of a deck of cards, or ½ to ¾ cup (125 mL to 185 mL) of flaked or canned fish.
- If you find it challenging to consistently eat 2 servings of higher-fat fish

each week, consider taking a daily fish oil capsule to ensure you are meeting your needs for this important fat. Most people should aim for about 300 to 500 milligrams of combined EPA and DHA a day (the label will tell you how many milligrams are in each capsule).

- If you already suffer from heart disease, take 1,000 milligrams (1 g) of combined EPA and DHA daily.
- If you suffer from high triglycerides, arthritis, or clinical depression, talk to your doctor before starting to supplement your diet with fish oil capsules. You may need to take 2,000 to 4,000 milligrams (2 to 4 g) of fish oil daily.

IS IT OKAY TO EAT SHELLFISH?

Yes! Shellfish—shrimp, crab, clams, oysters, lobster, mussels, and scallops—are low in fat, including unhealthy saturated fats, and rich in protein, iron, copper, zinc, and selenium. Although shrimp, lobster, and crab contain moderate amounts of cholesterol, they can easily fit into a healthy diet, especially if you don't drown them in butter!

GET MORE FISH IN YOUR EATING PLAN

Why don't people eat fish? Often they don't know how to cook or prepare it so that it tastes great. Don't let your lack of cooking savvy get in the way of enjoying omega-3-rich fish twice a week. Fish can and should be delicious. Try the salmon and rainbow trout recipes in this book,

FOOD *for* THOUGHT

"Omega-3 fatty acid levels in the blood have a greater impact on risk for heart disease than cholesterol, total fat, or fibre. The higher the omega-3 levels, the lower the risk of heart disease and death, and vice versa."

WILLIAM S. HARRIS, PHD, University of South Dakota

including Grilled Salmon with Mango Strawberry Salsa (page 227), Crumb-Topped Salmon with Parsley, Dill, and Lemon (page 235), and Rainbow Trout with Citrus, Ginger, and Fresh Thyme (page 237). Introduce your kids to fish early in life and serve it regularly. Enjoy fish when you dine out—and I'm not talking fish and chips or breaded fish sticks!

SHOULD I BUY FOODS THAT CONTAIN ADDED OMEGA-3 FATS?

An explosion of products fortified with omega-3 fats has flooded the market. Most contain relatively small amounts of these added fats and many contain plant source omega-3 fats (from flaxseeds or canola oil) rather than the most beneficial kinds of omega-3 fats found in fish and some algae (EPA and DHA). If you buy products with added omega-3 fats, look for those that list EPA or DHA on the label.

ENJOY FISH, BUT AVOID MERCURY

Limiting your exposure to mercury is important. It can accumulate in the body and cause substantial damage to your nervous system. To limit your intake, avoid bluefish, Chilean sea bass, escolar, grouper, mackerel (king and Spanish), marlin, orange roughy, sablefish, shark, swordfish, tilefish (also called golden bass or golden snapper), tuna steaks, and sushi made with tuna. Choose canned light tuna (made from skipjack tuna) rather than white (albacore) tuna, as it is much lower in mercury. If you prefer the taste of white (albacore) tuna, limit your intake to one serving (½ cup/125 mL) per week. Both wild and farmed salmon, rainbow trout, and sardines are great choices for omega-3 fats and are also low in mercury.

FISH OIL IS LOW IN MERCURY

Consumerlabs.com (which examined 41 fish oil products), Harvard University (which examined 5 popular brands of fish oil products), and Consumer Reports (which examined 16 fish oil products), concluded from their research that fish oil supplements are low in contaminants, including mercury.

LESSON LEARNED

Few foods protect health like the omega-3 fats found in fish. They reduce your risk of most diseases and provide especially powerful protection for your heart, brain, and eyes. They're also linked to a lower risk of depression. Eat 2 servings of higher-fat fish such as salmon or rainbow trout each week. If you don't eat fish regularly, consider taking a fish oil capsule that contains 300 to 500 mg of combined EPA and DHA. Avoid or limit fish that is high in mercury.

The Power of Green Tea

IN MOST CASES if food comes from a plant it's good for you. Tea is no exception. All true teas—which include white, green, oolong, and black teas as opposed to herbal teas—come from the same plant: *Camellia sinensis.* This plant is loaded with powerful, health-protective plant compounds called flavonoids that possess antioxidant, anti-inflammatory, anti-viral, and anti-bacterial properties. Each tea differs in the way it is processed. Both white tea (which comes from the young leaves of the plant) and green tea (which comes from the more mature leaves of the plant) are not fermented, which means their leaves are not exposed to air while drying. Oolong tea is partially fermented; black tea is fully fermented. Processing changes the antioxidant profile and potential health benefits of tea. While all four types of tea are good for your health, white and green teas are higher in antioxidants and provide more potent health protection.

PLENTY OF HEALTH BENEFITS

Tea, especially green tea, is linked to multiple health benefits, including a lower risk of heart disease, stroke, cancer, dementia, and type 2 diabetes. Research shows that tea is good for bone, eye, and dental health, including bad breath, tooth decay, and gum disease. It helps boost immunity and can ward off a cold or flu. If you drink tea, you may find it easier to maintain a healthy body weight (although what you eat and how much you exercise plays a far more significant role). Tea is even linked to an increase in endurance when exercising.

TEA DILATES YOUR ARTERIES

Regular tea drinkers have a lower risk of heart disease and stroke. The flavonoids in tea promote a healthy endothelium, which is the inner lining of all blood vessels. Researchers from the Netherlands reviewed nine studies looking at tea's ability to enhance flow-mediated dilation (a measure of a blood vessel's ability to expand or dilate). They found that drinking two to three cups of tea was linked to a 40% increase in artery diameter. Bottom line: A moderate consumption of tea substantially enhances the ability of the artery wall to relax and dilate, which may reduce your risk of heart disease and stroke.

TEA AND BRAIN HEALTH

The research on tea and brain health is exciting! Most studies have focused on green tea. The flavonoids in green tea help to prevent the formation and buildup of beta-amyloid in the brain. Beta-amyloid is a sticky, toxic protein that wraps around brain cells and destroys them, which leads to Alzheimer's. Green tea helps preserve overall learning and memory by protecting cells in the brain from damage and by chelating or removing iron, which reduces the formation of harmful free radicals. It has also been found to reduce brain cell death by impacting specific survival genes. In addition, there is strong evidence that drinking tea may lower risk of stroke. A stroke occurs when blood flow is interrupted to part of the brain. Stroke is the second leading cause of death, both in developed and developing countries, and a major cause of serious long-term disability worldwide. Bottom line: Take care of your brain and drink tea.

BETTER BRAIN FUNCTION AT 100

In the Chinese Longitudinal Healthy Longevity Survey, involving over 7,000 men and women between the ages of 80 and 115 years (average age 91), regular tea drinking was linked to better cognitive function. Daily tea drinkers had significantly higher verbal fluency scores than either occasional tea drinkers or non–tea drinkers.

TEA FIGHTS CANCER ALONG YOUR G.I. TRACT

Using data from the Shanghai Women's Health Study involving almost 70,000 women, researchers set out to determine if drinking tea was linked to a lower risk of digestive tract cancer, including cancers of the stomach, esophagus, and colon. They found that regular tea drinkers (those who consumed two to three cups daily, mostly green tea) cut their overall risk of these cancers by more than 20%. The reduction in risk increased as the amount and years of tea consumption increased. Women who had been drinking tea regularly for at least 20 years slashed their risk by almost 30%. The antioxidant flavonoids in tea may inhibit cancer by reducing damage to DNA as well as blocking tumour cell growth and invasion.

TEA FIGHTS SUPERBUGS

Antibiotic-resistant bacteria are a growing and deadly problem. Can green tea help? According to pharmacy researchers and members of the Society of General Microbiology, antibiotics may be up to three times more effective in their fight against resistant superbugs when taken with green tea. Twenty-eight disease-causing micro-organisms were tested. In every single case green tea enhanced the bacteria-killing activity of the antibiotics. Although further research is needed, it seems that tea is good for your immunity

FOOD *for* THOUGHT
"Better to be deprived of food for three days than tea for one."
ANCIENT CHINESE PROVERB

and demonstrates potent anti-viral and anti-bacterial actions.

HOW MUCH TEA SHOULD YOU DRINK?

You should drink about 3 to 6 cups of tea a day. This amount appears to provide good overall health protection and also keeps your intake of caffeine within a safe range. At this time the strongest research support is for green tea, although white tea also looks promising. All types of tea, however, including oolong and black tea, provide health benefits.

LIMIT CAFFEINE

The caffeine content of tea varies widely among brands of tea, as opposed to types of tea, and can range from 15 to 60 milligrams per cup—most contain about 40 milligrams per cup (250 mL). One small cup of coffee contains anywhere from about 80 to 175 milligrams of caffeine. Health Canada recommends that adults limit their intake of caffeine to 400 milligrams a day (no more than 300 milligrams during pregnancy). I don't recommend decaffeinated green or black tea because the decaffeination process destroys as much as 50% of the flavonoids (herbal teas are naturally caffeine-free). Caffeine, in moderation, fits into a healthy diet and even appears to provide further health protection (see page 66).

MAXIMIZING ANTIOXIDANTS

Research has found that about 85% of the antioxidants in tea are released within the first five minutes of brewing time. Take your tea with a squeeze of lemon rather than milk. Lemon juice and other foods that contain vitamin C have been found to increase the amount of flavonoids absorbed into the bloodstream as much as threefold.

A FEW NOTES OF CAUTION

- Don't drink your tea when it's very hot (160°F/70°C or higher) as this can damage your esophagus and increase your risk of esophageal cancer as much as eightfold. Researchers suggest waiting at least four minutes before drinking a cup of freshly boiled tea.
- Beware of bottled iced teas: Most are high in added sugar and very low in flavonoids. If you like iced tea, make it yourself and drink it the same day.
- Chai tea (spiced tea) can be healthy, especially if you make it yourself. I always add freshly sliced ginger, cinnamon sticks, and whole cloves to my daily pot of green tea. Beware of the chai tea found at your local coffee shop, however, as it may be loaded with sugar.

WHAT ABOUT HERBAL TEAS?

Herbal teas, such as chamomile, peppermint, and hibiscus, deserve a place in your daily diet alongside green or black teas, especially later in the day when you want to avoid caffeine. They also contain antioxidants and plant compounds that protect health.

Leave Room for Chocolate...
Especially Cocoa!

MY FIRST BOOK came out in 1998. It was called *When in Doubt, Eat Broccoli! (But Leave Some Room for Chocolate)* When I wrote that book I had no idea chocolate was going to become the superfood it is today. Does it deserve superstar status? Is it really worthy of a place in our daily diet? Here's what you need to know.

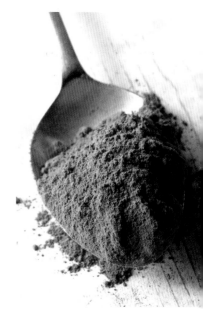

DRINK COCOA FOR A HEALTHY HEART

In the early 1990s, Harvard researchers began studying the Kuna Indians who live on small remote islands just off the coast of Panama. This population's rates of heart disease and stroke are among the lowest in the world. Cancer and type 2 diabetes are also uncommon. Most striking is the fact that their blood pressure does not increase with age, as seen in most other parts of the world. Those over the age of 60 have blood pressure that is as low as people in their twenties or thirties. How is this possible? The Kuna Indians drink about 4 to 5 cups of flavanol-rich cocoa each and every day. Flavanols are the plant compounds in cocoa and dark chocolate that are linked to good health. What happens when these people move to the mainland and stop drinking cocoa? They see dramatic increases in their blood pressure and experience a much higher risk

of disease—as much as 15 times higher. Cocoa appears to be an all-star protector of health.

HOW COCOA AND DARK CHOCOLATE KEEP US HEALTHY

Cocoa beans, from which cocoa and chocolate are made, are loaded (and I do mean *loaded*) with health-protective plant compounds called flavanols. Although these compounds are found in other foods like tea, red wine, apples, and berries, they are found in the highest concentration, by far, in the cocoa bean. Flavanols' greatest claim to fame are their ability to stimulate the release of nitric oxide in your body. Nitric oxide causes blood vessels to relax and widen, and improves blood flow to your heart, brain, muscles, and all your body parts. These compounds also reduce inflammation, decrease the stickiness of your blood (they have an aspirin-like effect), and act as potent antioxidants. They put cell-damaging free radicals that can lead to diseases such as cancer or dementia out of business.

COCOA PROMOTES GOOD BRAIN HEALTH

More and more research is showing that cocoa flavanols may keep your mind sharp. They boost blood flow to the brain and are linked to a lower risk of stroke and dementia. In a study from the University of L'Aquila in Italy involving 90 elderly men and women with mild cognitive impairment, those who consumed a daily flavanol-rich cocoa drink (containing about 500 milligrams of flavanols) for eight weeks saw significant improvement in their thinking and memory skills. In addition, blood pressure, resistance to insulin, and oxidative stress (which measures potential damage from free radicals) decreased.

CHOCOLATE FOR GOOD GUT HEALTH

The "good" or "friendly" bacteria that live along your gastrointestinal tract play a very important role in your health. Certain foods are considered "prebiotic," which means they provide a source of food for good bacteria to thrive and grow. In a study by the University of Reading in the UK involving 22 healthy volunteers, those who consumed a flavanol-rich cocoa beverage (494 milligrams of flavanols) every day for four weeks significantly increased the levels of the good bacteria in their colon.

NOT ALL CHOCOLATE IS CREATED EQUAL

Researchers from the Hershey Center for Health and Nutrition looked at the flavanol content of different chocolate products. On a gram weight basis, cocoa powder has the highest flavanol concentration followed by (from most to least) unsweetened baking chocolate, dark chocolate (including semi-sweet baking chips), milk chocolate, and chocolate syrup. White chocolate does not contain any flavanols (it's not made with cocoa solids).

WHAT TYPE OF COCOA IS BEST?

Avoid "Dutch-processed" cocoa that has been treated with an alkalizing agent such as baking soda (it will say potassium carbonate or sodium carbonate on the ingredient label). This is done to reduce the acidity and mellow the flavour of cocoa, but it results in a loss of 40% to as much as 90% of flavanols. Hershey's and Ghirardelli are just two of the companies that produce "natural" cocoa products—they are your best choice. When you bake with cocoa, be sure to add both baking powder and baking soda to help preserve the flavanols.

WHAT KIND OF CHOCOLATE IS BEST?

In most cases, the more cocoa a chocolate product contains, the higher its flavanol content. It's wise to choose dark chocolate over milk chocolate and to look for a bar that contains at least 60% to 70% cocoa. However, significant flavanol losses can take place during cocoa bean processing, especially in the roasting and fermentation stages of production, so it pays to do some research before buying a product. Some companies, including Mars (CocoaVia and Dove Dark), Hershey's (Special Dark and Extra Dark), and Callebaut (Acticoa), process their cocoa and chocolate products in such a way as to minimize such losses. In the future, we may see the flavanol content of all chocolate products listed on package labels. I would fully endorse it!

MORE REASONS TO KEEP IT DARK

I always recommend dark chocolate over milk chocolate. Not only does dark chocolate provide greater health protection, most people are much more likely to over-indulge in milk chocolate. Research from the University of Copenhagen in Denmark also reports that dark chocolate is significantly more filling than milk chocolate. Keep it dark!

GET MORE COCOA
IN YOUR EATING PLAN

Getting at least 200 milligrams of cocoa flavanols daily may help you maintain the elasticity of your blood vessels. Higher intake, closer to 500 milligrams daily, may provide even greater health protection.

Ongoing research will tell us more. One tablespoon (15 mL) of natural cocoa powder contains about 150 to 175 milligrams of flavanols. Cocoa is also very low in fat and calories (just 10 calories per 1 tablespoon/15 mL). It is by far the healthiest way to get more flavanols into your diet. You can stir cocoa into coffee (or lattes or cappuccino), milk, yogurt, oatmeal, or shakes. Be sure to try my Spiced Cocoa Banana Smoothie (page 237).

As for dark chocolate, the flavanol content varies considerably depending on cocoa content and processing. One ounce (28 g or about four squares) of most dark chocolate contains about 65 to 75 milligrams of flavanols. Dark chocolate that has a high cocoa content and has been processed to preserve flavanols, however, may contain as much as 180 milligrams per ounce or more. This same amount of chocolate, however, also comes with about 150 calories, 9 grams of fat, and 3 teaspoons (15 mL) of sugar. That's why limiting chocolate to no more than about 1 ounce a day (28 g or about four squares) makes sense for most people (unless you lead a very active lifestyle and can afford the extra calories). Cocoa is the best way to up your intake of flavanols.

LESSON LEARNED

Cocoa beans are loaded with plant compounds called flavanols that provide potent health protection, especially for your heart and blood vessels. Enjoy dark chocolate (at least 60% to 70% cocoa) in small amounts (no more than about 1 ounce/28 grams daily). The healthiest way to get more flavanols into your diet is by consuming natural cocoa.

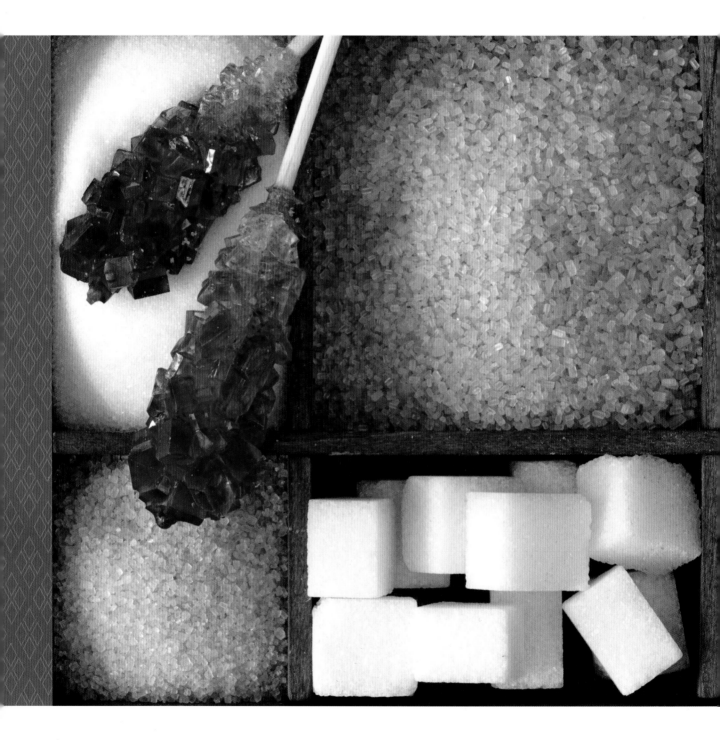

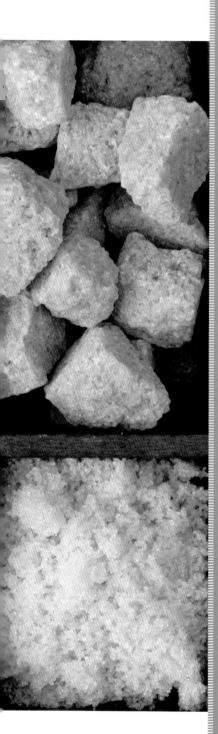

DIETARY VILLAINS AND OTHER HEALTH HAZARDS

Dining Out Can Harm Your Health

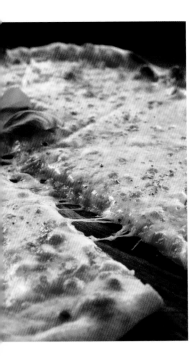

MOST OF US lead busy lives. Dining out can be an enjoyable and convenient way to feed our families and ourselves. Where you dine, how often you dine, and what you dine on, however, can greatly damage your health and your waistline. Here is what you need to know:

THE TRUTH ABOUT DINING OUT

- Most people greatly underestimate how harmful a restaurant or fast-food meal can be. Most meals outside the home come loaded with far more calories, sodium, unhealthy fats, and sugar than you need.
- Fast-food meals, in particular, are usually lacking in fruits, vegetables, and milk, as well as valuable nutrients like vitamin C, calcium, iron, and fibre. People are also more likely to consume sugary drinks with these meals.
- Although most fast-food restaurants now carry at least some healthy items, people often don't buy them.
- The frequency with which many people dine out, including busy families and especially teens, is dangerous to health. The risk of heart disease, type 2 diabetes, and obesity all go up.
- Every fast-food meal you consume increases your risk of being overweight. Eating two to three fast-food meals per week is linked to as much as a 60% to 80% greater risk of obesity. No other lifestyle factor is so strongly linked to severe obesity than the consumption of fast food.
- Convenience stores significantly contribute to the number of unhealthy food items consumed each day.

FAST FOOD IS HARMFUL TO HEALTH

What happens when a population that normally doesn't eat fast food starts consuming it? Researchers from the University of Minnesota School of Public Health studied the eating habits of over 52,000 men and women in Singapore over a 16-year period starting in 1993 (when fast-food restaurants entered their local food environment for the first time). The results were not pretty. Those people who consumed fast food two or more times per week increased their risk of dying from heart disease by more than 50% and their risk of developing type 2 diabetes by almost 30%. Eating fast food four or more times a week was linked to an almost 80% increase in heart disease. Bottom line: Fast-food restaurants are not good for a country or the people who live there!

JUST ONE FAST-FOOD MEAL DAMAGES ARTERIES

Researchers from the University of Montreal report that consuming a single fast-food meal high in saturated fat damages arteries, while no damage occurs after consuming a Mediterranean-style meal rich in healthy fats. After eating the fast-food meal, the arteries of the study participants (28 non-smoking men) dilated 24% less than when in the fasting state. In contrast, the arteries dilated normally and maintained good blood flow after the Mediterranean-style meal. Poor endothelial function (measured by the ability of the artery to dilate) is one of the most significant precursors of heart disease.

SAVE YOUR LIVER

Strong evidence suggests that a diet high in fast food can be toxic to your liver. Liver specialists, however, say that you can undo this damage if you change your habits, start eating healthy, and stay physically active. If you don't, you're looking for trouble. Doctors are starting to see children and teens with cirrhosis of the liver, a serious disease normally seen in adults with a history of alcohol abuse or hepatitis C. These kids are consuming too many calories, too much fat, and too much sugar from unhealthy foods. Something has to change!

WORKING PARENTS LISTEN UP!

In many households both mom and dad need to head out the door to work each day. Unfortunately, this has repercussions on both our health and our children's health. A study by Temple University in Boston involving almost 4,000 parents found that when women work full-time the result is fewer family meals, less frequent encouragement of their adolescents' healthful eating, lower fruit and vegetable intakes, and less time spent on food preparation. If either parent has a high-stress job, intakes of both sugar-sweetened drinks and fast food typically go up, as does the risk of their children becoming obese. Other research by Cornell University in New York suggests that fathers who work long hours are more likely to order take-out, miss family meals, purchase prepared entrées, and eat while working.

Mealtime Tips for Busy Parents:

- Dedicate time to food planning, food shopping, and advance meal preparation in the evenings and on weekends.
- Make bigger batches of food to freeze for future meals, take for lunches, and use for leftovers.
- Grab healthy take-out options on the way home, such as veggie platters, fruit trays, pre-made salads (including bean salads), sushi, and rotisserie-cooked chicken (remove the skin).
- Get dads more involved in food

> **FOOD *for* THOUGHT**
> "Everybody knows that fast food is bad for you, but people continue to eat it because it tastes good. We're genetically programmed to prefer high-calorie foods, and sadly fast-food chains will continue to sell unhealthy foods because it earns them a living."
> **DARREL FRANCIS, MD,** National Heart and Lung Institute, Imperial College London

shopping and cooking (Cornell University research shows they're not doing as much as they could).

- Teach your kids to cook so they can fend for themselves and help prepare family meals.

THE BOTTOM LINE Plan ahead, stay organized, and make healthy meals a priority for you and your family.

SLOW DOWN

Fast food is called "fast" for a reason: It's fast to order and fast to eat. Speed and eating, however, don't go well together. Researchers from Osaka University in Japan looked at the eating habits of over 3,200 men and women. Those people who said they "ate until full and quickly" were three times more likely to be overweight than those who said they "ate until full and did not eat quickly." When you slow your eating, you give your body time to register all the calories you just consumed. Bottom line: People who eat slower eat less.

RESTAURANT MEALS CONTAIN UP TO THREE TIMES AS MANY CALORIES AS NEEDED

Researchers from Tufts University in Boston analyzed meals frequently purchased from independent and small-chain restaurants that generally don't post nutritional information about their menu items. They looked at 157 full meals from 33 different restaurants, including Mexican, American, Chinese, Italian, Japanese, Thai, Indian, Greek, and Vietnamese. On average, the meals contained 1,327 calories. This is about two to three times more calories than the average person should eat at one meal. Among the types of meals studied, the Italian (1,755 calories), American (1,494 calories), and Chinese (1,474 cal-ories) meals had the highest average calorie levels. Vietnamese meals had the lowest levels (922 calories), followed by Japanese (1,027 calories). Some meals contained over 2,000 calories per meal—more than you should have in an entire day! Bottom line: Restaurant meals generally contain an insane amount of calories.

PORTION DISTORTION

Do you suffer from portion distortion? Many people do. You can get so used to seeing large portions that they start seeming "normal." Most restaurant portions are two to five times larger than recommended for good health. Research consistently shows that the more food we're served, the more food we eat, even when our intention is to do otherwise. Take leftovers home to eat for lunch the next day. Share appetizers, share the main course, and if you order dessert, share that, too!

WHERE ARE THE CALORIES COMING FROM?

Since the 1970s, calorie consumption has been increasing, and waistlines have been expanding. Researchers from the University of North Carolina wanted to determine what factors contributed most to these changes. They found that both an increase in eating and drinking occasions (number of meals and snacks) and an increase in portion size were most strongly to blame. Bottom line: We're eating too often and too much!

LOSE THE WEIGHT AND KEEP IT OFF

Let's assume you've successfully lost the weight you wanted to lose. How do you make sure you don't gain it back? Researchers from the Centers for Disease Control and Prevention in Atlanta looked at what factors were associated with successful weight maintenance. They found that men and women were more likely to achieve success if they:

- ate at least 5 servings of fruits and vegetables daily
- engaged in at least 150 minutes or more of physical activity per week (for example, exercising for at least 30 minutes five days a week)
- shared portions when dining out
- avoided fast-food restaurants

In contrast, those who ate at fast-food restaurants two or more times per week were significantly more likely to regain the weight they had lost.

BUFFET RESTAURANTS AND OVERINDULGENCE

Everything about a buffet screams "eat more than you need!" The food options are endless, tempting you at every turn. You can refill your plate as many times as you wish. You don't get charged more if you eat more (getting your money's worth is important!). The dessert options alone are enough to put you well over your daily calorie allotment. The bottom line: Don't eat at buffet restaurants unless you have amazing self-control and know how to choose wisely. Otherwise, do so at your own peril. Buffet restaurants and overeating simply go hand in hand. Eating more calories than you need is pretty much a guarantee!

LESSON LEARNED

When dining out most people consume far more calories, fat, sodium, and sugar than they need. Frequent dining out, especially fast-food dining, greatly increases the risk of heart disease, type 2 diabetes, and obesity. Dine at home more often, and when dining out, be wise and choose well.

Making Better Choices
When Dining Out

FOOD *for* THOUGHT

"Limit yourself to no more than one fast-food meal a week. For some people, that's going to be a major downshift. But for the sake of your health, a visit to a fast-food restaurant should be considered a treat— not a regular event."

BRENT TETRI, MD, PROFESSOR, Saint Louis University Liver Center

I F YOU ARE going to dine out, you have to be mindful and make wise choices, otherwise your waistline and your health will pay the consequences. Here's my advice to help you on your way.

CHOOSE:

- Many places, including coffee shops like Starbucks, offer oatmeal with dried fruit, nuts, or berries. This is one of the healthiest menu options offered and a good choice any time of day.
- I am a huge fan of salads, including main-course salads, especially when they are made with nutritious ingredients like dark leafy greens and a healthy source of protein (nuts, beans, grilled chicken, or fish). All salads, however, can be high in calories and fat, and many are loaded with sodium. The dressing is usually the culprit. Ask that your salad be lightly dressed or request the dressing on the side. Watch out for unhealthy extras like croutons, bacon bits, and cheese.
- Bagels are usually a healthier choice over most muffins or donuts. Stick with 100% whole-grain varieties and consider sharing with a friend (most bagels are the equivalent of three slices of bread). Whenever you dine out, always look for 100% whole-grain options, including breads, pasta, tortillas, and brown rice.
- Fajitas and stir-fries made with lots of veggies and lean protein (such as chicken or shrimp) are healthier than many other menu items, although most still contain more sodium than recommended. Portions, especially for fajitas, can easily be divided in two.
- Grilled fish or chicken (skinless) with a side of veggies are good entrée options. If you go for steak, sirloin steak and filet mignon are leanest— just remember that most steaks are two to four times larger than you need.
- Yogurt berry or fruit parfaits (small size) are generally a healthy snack. They are relatively low in calories and contain good nutrition. Low-fat frozen yogurt mixed with fresh fruit is another good option.

AVOID OR LIMIT

- Be careful when ordering sandwiches. While a very small wrap may contain less than 300 calories, a large panini can contain over 1,000 calories and a huge dose of sodium. Go for smaller sandwiches made with whole-grain breads, lots of veggies, and lean protein. Limit fatty meats, such as salami or bacon, high-fat condiments, and cheese.

- If you love pizza (who doesn't!), go for multi-grain, thin-crust pizza and top with lots of veggies. Limit yourself to two slices.

- If you enjoy a good burger now and again, choose child-size portions or share your burger with a friend. Load your burger with shredded lettuce and tomatoes, not bacon and cheese.

- At many restaurants the appetizers are calorie disasters waiting to happen. Nachos, garlic cheese bread, and anything battered or deep-fried have more calories, fat, and sodium than the main meal. If you want an appetizer, stick to something small and healthy such as a small side salad (easy on the dressing).

- Stay away from wings, poutine, ribs, giant burgers, and pasta with cream sauces (or eat them only on your birthday!). They are the most unhealthy offenders for your body and your waistline.

- Most pasta meals are very high in calories, fat, and sodium due to the large portion sizes. A reasonable serving of pasta is no more than about 1½ cups (375 mL). If you order pasta, share it with a friend or take some home. Tomato-based sauces generally contain less fat and calories, but they're still high in sodium.

- Most people are consuming far too many calories in liquid form. Stay away from specialty coffees loaded with unhealthy syrups, sugar, and whipped cream. Stick with tea or coffee, or perhaps a latte or cappuccino sprinkled with cinnamon and nutmeg.

- Store-bought or restaurant smoothies can also be high in calories and in added sugar. Homemade smoothies are generally a better choice.

- Do I even have to tell you not to drink sugar-sweetened soft drinks? Don't. The same goes for other sugar-loaded beverages, such as iced tea and lemonade. Among the worst items on most menus are the shakes or blended ice-cream drinks—many contain 1,000 calories or more! Drink water, milk, or even a small chocolate milk instead.

- Most people don't need dessert. Go for a walk instead.

LESSON LEARNED

When dining out choose healthier options, including oatmeal, yogurt, salads (lightly dressed), whole grains, lean protein, and lots of veggies. Watch out for calorie-laden appetizers, giant burgers, pizza, ribs, wings, too much pasta, and calorie-loaded drinks, including specialty coffees, soft drinks, and even smoothies.

Sitting Is the New Smoking...
Get Off Your Butt!

LESSON LEARNED

Your body was not meant to sit for long periods of time. It's harmful to health and can kill you. Minimize the damage by walking 2 minutes for every 20 to 30 minutes of sitting time.

PROLONGED SITTING—WHETHER AT a computer, in front of the television, or in your car—is not just bad for your health, it's deadly. Researchers say the evidence is strong enough to support doctors prescribing the following to their patients: reduce daily sitting time!

SITTING KILLS

Research from the University of Western Sydney in Australia involving over 63,000 men aged 45 to 64 found that men who sat for more than four hours a day were significantly more likely to report having a chronic disease such as cancer, diabetes, heart disease, and high blood pressure. As time spent sitting increased, so did the risk of disease. Other research from the same university involving over 200,000 men and women found that inactive people who sat the most had double the risk of dying within three years compared with active people who sat the least.

The University of Leicester in the UK analyzed 18 studies involving almost 800,000 people and found that those who spend most of their day sitting are 147% more likely to suffer a heart attack or stroke, and 90% more likely to die from it if they do. Diabetes risk goes up by 112%. The chance of premature death jumps by about 50%. Other research has found a link between sitting and cancer risk, including cancer of the colon.

WHY IS SITTING SO DEADLY?

The human body was not designed to sit—not for long periods of time. It totally rebels when you do: Inflammation increases. Your resistance to insulin goes up (a key risk factor for diabetes development). Fat begins to accumulate around your belly. You're more likely to experience unhealthy blood cholesterol levels as well as high blood pressure. If you think starting or ending your day with a good workout or a long walk is the answer, it's not. While regular physical activity is critical to good health and should not be missed, too much sitting is a separate risk factor all on its own. The solution: Stand up and walk 2 minutes for every 20 to 30 minutes of sitting time (dancing or jumping around is also an option). Set a timer if you have to. When you take small breaks from sitting, it helps to lessen the harm of a sedentary day. It helps give your body what it wants and needs. Your body wants to move!

If I Told You Salt Could Kill You, Would You Eat Less of It?

WHY LOWER YOUR sodium (salt) intake? There is overwhelming scientific evidence that salt is a major cause of high blood pressure and that eating less salt lowers blood pressure. High blood pressure leads to heart attacks, strokes, heart failure, and kidney failure. The World Health Organization considers it the leading risk factor for death in the world.

EVERYONE BENEFITS FROM LESS SODIUM

Researchers from Queen Mary University of London reviewed 34 studies involving over 3,000 men and women to determine the effects of salt reduction on blood pressure. They found that a modest reduction in salt intake for four or more weeks causes significant and important falls in blood pressure in both those with normal and high blood pressure, regardless of gender or ethnic group. They found that the greater the reduction in salt intake, the greater the fall in blood pressure, and concluded that the results provide strong support for a reduction in population-wide salt intake.

REDUCING SALT SAVES LIVES

In the 1970s, Finland began a salt-reduction campaign. The population's average consumption of salt fell by about one-third over 30 years. During the same period, average blood pressure fell significantly (the population average fell more than 10 mmHg) and there was a 75% to 80% decrease in death from both stroke and heart disease. Sounds like a successful campaign to me!

LESS SODIUM, MORE POTASSIUM

Potassium is a nutrient most people don't get enough of. Sodium increases blood pressure; potassium lowers it. To get enough potassium, consume a diet rich in beans, nuts, low-fat milk, and yogurt. Load up on the fruits and vegetables, especially those that are dark green and orange.

SODIUM ALERT: PIZZA

Teenagers consume, on average, twice as much sodium as they should and more sodium than any other age group. Research from the University of California suggests that reducing salt in teenagers' diets could significantly reduce their risk of heart disease in adulthood. Pizza is the number-one source of sodium in the diet of many young adults.

> FOOD *for* THOUGHT
> "The single most dangerous ingredient in the food supply is salt."
> **CENTER FOR SCIENCE IN THE PUBLIC INTEREST, WASHINGTON, D.C.**

LESSON LEARNED

Most people consume too much sodium. Excess sodium leads to high blood pressure, which is lethal. It causes heart attacks, strokes, heart failure, and kidney failure. Aim for no more than about 1,500 milligrams of sodium a day (about two-thirds of a teaspoon of salt).

ARE YOU SALT-SENSITIVE?

Is it true that some people are more sensitive to the blood pressure raising effect of sodium than others? Yes. African Americans, people who already suffer from high blood pressure (including a large percentage of the population who are overweight and sedentary), and middle-aged and older adults tend to be more salt-sensitive. Everyone, however, benefits by putting down the salt shaker. In addition to causing blood pressure to go up, a high-salt diet may increase your risk of stomach cancer, hardening of the arteries, and kidney stones, and is bad for bone health.

SALT, KIDNEY STONES, AND BONE HEALTH

Researchers from the University of Alberta recently discovered an important link between sodium and calcium: They both appear to be regulated by the same molecule in the body. When sodium intake becomes too high, the body gets rid of sodium via urine, taking calcium with it, which depletes calcium stores in the body. High levels of calcium in the urine lead to the development of kidney stones, while inadequate levels of calcium in the body lead to thin bones and osteoporosis. In research from Shimane University in Japan involving over 200 post-menopausal women, a high-salt diet increased the risk of breaking a bone fourfold, even in those with higher bone density.

HOW MUCH SODIUM DO WE REALLY NEED?

The human body requires only a small amount of sodium and is very efficient at conserving what it needs. The Yanomamo people inhabit the forests of the Amazon in Brazil. They take in just 200 milligrams of sodium daily, which is 17 times less sodium than found in the typical North American diet. High blood pressure is virtually absent in their society.

RECOMMENDED SODIUM INTAKE

In 2004, the Institute of Medicine released its official recommendation for sodium, stating that most adults should aim to consume no more than about 1,500 milligrams of sodium a day (1 tsp/ 5 mL of salt contains about 2,300 milligrams of sodium). This is consistent with current guidelines from the American Heart Association. More recently (May 2013), the Institute of Medicine relaxed its guidelines, stating that limiting sodium to 2,300 milligrams daily is sufficient for most people. In Canada and the United States, most people average about 3,400 milligrams of sodium daily (about 1½ tsp/7 mL of salt). Bottom line: No matter which guideline you go by, most of us consume significantly more sodium than is good for health and well-being. I believe aiming closer to the 1,500 milligram guideline is best for overall health. Our food supply in its natural state contains only small amounts of sodium.

Top 10 Tips to Reduce Your Sodium Intake

TO PROTECT YOUR health and reduce your risk of high blood pressure, here are 10 great ways to reduce the amount of sodium in your eating plan:

1. To limit sodium to no more than 1,500 milligrams a day (based on eating three meals and two snacks), aim for about 400 to 500 milligrams of sodium per meal and about 100 to 200 milligrams or less of sodium per snack.

2. Always read food labels and enjoy more home-cooked meals that are healthier and lower in sodium. As much as 80% of the sodium most people consume comes from packaged processed food and restaurant meals.

3. Limit dining out (just one fast-food or restaurant meal can contain two to three days' worth of sodium). When you do go out for fast food, go online before you dine and choose healthier, lower-sodium fare. In restaurants, ask that foods be prepared without added salt and season your food yourself, sensibly.

4. Foods labelled "reduced in sodium" can still be loaded with salt. A "sodium-reduced" product must contain at least

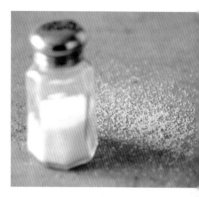

25% less sodium than the regular product. Some products, such as soy sauce, are so high in salt to begin with that even sodium-reduced varieties contain as much as 600 milligrams of sodium per 1 tablespoon (15 mL).

5. Look for food labels that say "salt-free" (less than 5 milligrams of sodium per serving) or "low in sodium" (140 milligrams of sodium or less per serving). Remember that the amount of sodium contained in different brands of the same food item can vary as much as tenfold. Always compare products and choose lower-sodium brands.

6. Know where the sodium in your diet is coming from, so it is easier to cut back. For most people, a significant amount of sodium comes from eating breads, rolls, and cereals. We also get a lot of sodium from processed meats (cold cuts, bacon, sausages, hot dogs), soups, tomato-based foods (tomato juice, tomato sauce, salsa), pizza, processed

pasta and rice dishes (macaroni and cheese or rice mixtures with added seasonings), cheese, snack foods (chips, pretzels, popcorn), frozen dinners, sauces, marinades, and salad dressings. Choose carefully when buying any of these products and/or eat less of them.

7. Buy vegetables that are fresh, frozen, or canned "with no salt added." Buy fresh fish, poultry, and lean meat rather than canned, breaded, or processed products. Rinse canned foods, such as beans or tuna, to remove some of the sodium and look for brands with "no salt added."

8. Take the salt shaker off the table. Make it available only upon request and never add salt without first tasting your food. Too many people reach for the salt shaker out of habit. When cooking with salt, add it late in the cooking process so the other ingredients in your dish have time to release their flavours—you'll be less likely to over-salt your food.

9. Learn to cook and prepare foods with onions, garlic, herbs, spices, lemon

and lime juice or zest, flavoured vinegars or oils, peppers, and salt-free seasoning blends (such as Mrs. Dash) instead of salt.

10. Reduce your sodium intake gradually, over a period of 8 to 12 weeks. If you think you can't get used to eating less salt, research says otherwise. Although scientists believe we're born with a preference for salty flavour, good evidence shows the amount of salt we like is learned. Teens who frequently eat fast food, for example, develop a preference for salty foods. We can learn to accept and enjoy foods that contain less sodium.

IS SEA SALT HEALTHIER?

The only reason to use sea salt over regular salt is because you prefer the taste and ideally use less of it. Both types of salt, however, are a significant source of sodium and, in excess, can harm your health. Some sea salts may contain small amounts of trace minerals, but they may not contain iodine, an essential nutrient added to table salt. Iodine is necessary for proper functioning of the thyroid gland.

LESSON LEARNED

To cut back on sodium, limit intake to about 400 to 500 milligrams per meal and 100 to 200 milligrams per snack. Read food labels, compare brands, eat unprocessed food, limit fast-food and restaurant dining, and learn to season your food without salt.

Sugar

WAISTLINE EXPANDER, EMPTY CALORIE CONTRIBUTOR, AND DISEASE PROMOTER

NORTH AMERICANS CONSUME as much as 20 to 30 teaspoons (100 to 150 mL) of sugar daily. That's a crazy amount of sugar! Major sources are sugar-sweetened drinks (soft drinks, energy drinks, sports drinks, fruit drinks, specialty coffees or teas, and sweetened bottled waters), grain desserts (cakes, cookies, donuts, pies, granola bars), dairy desserts (ice cream, frozen yogurt, shakes), candy, and cold cereals. Here's what you need to know.

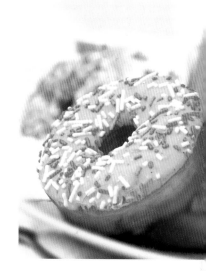

WHAT'S THE DOWNSIDE OF ALL THIS SUGAR?

- Sugary diets may increase heart-disease risk by increasing triglycerides and blood pressure and by creating an inflammatory environment in the body. High-sugar foods like soft drinks are also linked to a higher risk of obesity, type 2 diabetes, pancreatic cancer, gout, and fatty liver disease.

- Sugar provides no nutritional value other than calories—calories that most of us don't want or need and that can contribute to obesity.

- High-sugar foods often replace more nutritious foods. As sugar intake goes up, our intake of many vitamins and minerals goes down.

- The frequent consumption of sugar-laden foods can cause tooth decay and gum disease.

THE SUGAR–DIABETES CONNECTION

Researchers from Stanford University in California looked at data on sugar availability and diabetes rates from 175 countries over the past decade. They found that for every additional 150 calories of sugar available per person per day (the amount found in one regular can of soft drink), the prevalence of diabetes in the population rose 1.1%, even after taking into consideration other risk factors such as obesity, physical activity, other types of calories, and a number of economic and social variables. This link was not found with any other type of food. The longer a population was exposed to excess sugar, the higher the rate of diabetes.

HOW SUGAR HARMS YOUR HEART

Based on data from the National Health and Nutrition Examination Survey involving over 6,000 US adults, those who got 10% or more of their calories from added sugars (about 14 teaspoons/70 mL daily) were significantly more likely to have low levels of HDL (good) cholesterol and higher levels of triglycerides—both risk factors for the development of heart disease. The risk of low HDL levels was as much as 300% greater in people who ate more sugar.

TOO MUCH SUGAR IS BAD FOR YOUR BRAIN

Researchers from the Mayo Clinic tracked the eating habits of over 1,200 people ages 70 to 89 over four years. People with the highest sugar intake were 1.5 times more likely to experience mild cognitive impairment, including problems with memory, language, thinking, and judgment, than those with the lowest sugar intakes.

SUGAR AND EXPANDING WAISTLINES

Want to lose weight? Cut back on sugar. That's the conclusion of researchers from the University of Otago in New Zealand. They reviewed 71 studies and found that cutting back on sugar results in significant weight loss, while increasing sugar intake results in significant weight gain. Makes sense to me.

EVEN BABIES ARE GETTING TOO MUCH

In a Canadian study funded by the Centre for Science in the Public Interest, more than half (53%) of foods targeted to toddlers in Canadian grocery stores were found to contain an excessive amount of sugar. The study examined 186 foods marketed specifically for babies and toddlers, excluding fruit and vegetable purées. Is it necessary to add so much sugar to these baby and toddler products in the first place? No. It only promotes a love for sugar at an early age.

HOW MUCH ADDED SUGAR IS HEALTHY?

The term "added sugars" refers to sugars and syrups you add to foods, as well as sugars and syrups that are added to processed foods. This includes white sugar, brown sugar, honey, and maple syrup. It does not include the sugar that occurs naturally in foods such as fruit, milk, and plain yogurt (milk sugar). The most recent guidelines come from the American Heart Association. They recommend the following limit for added sugars:

WOMEN   6 teaspoons (30 mL) daily (based on 1,800 calorie diet)

MEN   9 teaspoons (45 mL) daily (based on 2,200 calorie diet)

Although no official recommendation exists for children, based on these recommendations most young children (ages four to nine) should have no more than about 5 teaspoons (25 mL) of added sugar daily.

LABEL-READING TIP

To determine how many teaspoons of sugar a product contains, divide the grams of "sugars" listed on the food label by four. For example, if a granola bar contains 12 grams of sugars, that translates to 3 teaspoons (15 mL) of sugar per bar.

HOW CAN YOU TELL IF A PRODUCT CONTAINS ADDED SUGAR, NOT JUST NATURALLY OCCURRING SUGAR?

Look for sugar on the ingredient list. It can appear in many different forms and may be listed as:

- agave syrup
- beet sugar
- cane sugar
- corn sweetener
- corn syrup
- dextrose
- evaporated cane juice
- fructose
- fruit juice concentrates
- glucose
- high-fructose corn syrup
- honey
- invert sugar
- malt syrup
- maltose
- maple syrup
- molasses
- raw sugar
- sucrose
- turbinado sugar

Be especially careful to avoid products that list sugar as the first or second ingredient on the label.

"REAL FRUIT" GUMMIES?

Many kids love processed fruit-leather and fruit-gummy snacks. The labels say they're made with 100% real fruit. Are they a good choice? Although some offer small amounts of nutrition, for the most part they're fruit imposters. Most are made primarily with "fruit juice concentrates," which means sugar and not much else. If you want your kids to eat fruit, give them whole, real fruit. Dried fruit, like dried apricots, is also a better choice than fruit snacks made with fruit juice concentrates.

IS DRIED FRUIT GOOD FOR YOU?

Yes, dried fruit is good for you in small quantities. When fruits are dried and the water is removed, they generally become more concentrated in vitamins, minerals, fibre, and antioxidants. The antioxidant content of dates and prunes (dried plums), for example, rivals berries. Water-soluble nutrients like vitamin C, however, are lost during processing, and dried fruit is also very concentrated in sugar and calories. Limit yourself to no more than about one serving (¼ cup/60 mL) a day.

HOW TO REDUCE YOUR SUGAR INTAKE

- Satisfy your sweet tooth with fresh fruit. Limit 100% fruit juice to 1 cup (250 mL) daily. Stay away from "fruit drinks" and "fruit beverages"—most contain primarily sugar and water.
- Avoid or limit sugar-sweetened beverages including soft drinks, energy drinks, sports drinks, shakes, specialty coffees, and some smoothies.
- Avoid or limit high-sugar, nutrient-poor foods like candy and desserts.
- Buy plain yogurt and add your own fruit.

FOOD *for* THOUGHT
"Which is worse, the sugar or the fat? The sugar, a thousand times over."
DR. ROBERT LUSTIG,
University of California

- Buy unsweetened cereal and sweeten with dried or fresh fruit.
- Season your food with sweet spices, including cinnamon, nutmeg, and allspice.

HOW BAD IS HIGH-FRUCTOSE CORN SYRUP?

High-fructose corn syrup and white table sugar (sucrose) are both made up of almost equal parts glucose and fructose. They contain the same number of calories, possess the same level of sweetness, and are absorbed through the gastrointestinal tract in the exact same way. The bottom line: All kinds of sugar harm health when consumed in excess.

ARE SOME TYPES OF SUGAR OR SWEETENERS HEALTHIER THAN OTHERS?

Molasses is the most nutritious sugar. Dark honey (like buckwheat, manuka, blueberry, and eucalyptus) and real maple syrup contain plant compounds called polyphenols that may have health benefits. Agave nectar has a lower glycemic index than most other sugars (the sugar it contains is released more slowly into the bloodstream). Fruit sugars, like date sugar, can be high in antioxidants. The bottom line: More natural sugars are a better choice, but must still be consumed in small amounts to protect health.

DO SUGAR SUBSTITUTES MAKE SENSE?

Sugar substitutes or low-calorie sweeteners like stevia, sucralose (Splenda), and aspartame (Equal or NutraSweet), in moderation, can help reduce sugar and calorie intake. Stevia appears to be the safest and most natural sweetener. Learning to enjoy foods with less sweetness and foods that are naturally sweet, such as fruit, is your healthiest option.

LESSON LEARNED

Sugar is bad for health and most of us eat way too much of it. It's linked to a higher risk of many diseases, including heart disease, diabetes, and obesity. Most women should aim for no more than 6 teaspoons (30 mL) of added sugar daily; men no more than 9 teaspoons (45 mL) daily. To limit sugar, read food labels and avoid high-sugar foods like soft drinks.

Why You Should *not* Drink Regular Soft Drinks

ON'T DRINK SUGAR-SWEETENED soft drinks or pop. Don't have them in your home. Soft drinks are called "liquid candy" for good reason. They're loaded with sugar: one can (12 oz/355 mL) contains about 10 teaspoons (50 mL). They also provide no nutritional value and often take the place of healthier options. Compared with 30 years ago, our consumption of soft drinks has tripled. They are a leading source of calories and sugar in many people's diets. Some researchers believe they're so detrimental to health that they should carry warning labels similar to those seen on cigarette packages. Drinking just 1 to 2 servings a day can damage your health and increase your risk of disease.

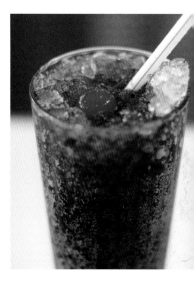

REGULAR SOFT DRINK CONSUMERS MAY BE MORE LIKELY TO SUFFER FROM:

- OBESITY no other food or drink has a stronger link to obesity
- TYPE 2 DIABETES a nasty disease, with even nastier complications if not managed
- GESTATIONAL DIABETES the type of diabetes that develops during pregnancy
- METABOLIC SYNDROME a group of risk factors that includes high blood pressure, high blood sugar, unhealthy blood fats, and abdominal obesity
- GOUT an acute form of arthritis that causes severe pain and swelling in the joints; most commonly affects the big toe, but may also affect the heel, ankle, hand, wrist, or elbow

- FATTY LIVER fat accumulates in the liver causing inflammation and scarring; can progress to liver failure
- KIDNEY STONES stones originate in the kidney and pass into the urinary tract; can be extremely painful
- PANCREATIC CANCER one of the deadliest cancers

88 STUDIES CAN'T BE WRONG!

Yale University researchers reviewed 88 studies and found, not surprisingly, that soft drinks are bad for health. They are linked to an increase in calories; a higher body weight; lower intakes of milk, calcium, and other nutrients; and an increase in type 2 diabetes. Their conclusion: The science strongly supports recommendations to reduce the consumption of soft drinks.

FOOD *for* THOUGHT

"Sugar-sweetened beverages—avoid, avoid, avoid!"

RACHEL JOHNSON,
Nutrition Professor,
University of Vermont

JUST ONE DAMAGES HEALTH

Research from Imperial College London involving over 27,000 participants from eight different European countries revealed that drinking just one soft drink (12 oz/355 mL) a day was enough to raise the risk of type 2 diabetes by 22%.

KIDNEY STONES GIVE NEW MEANING TO THE WORD "PAIN"

Kidney stones can be excruciating painful. Many people describe the pain as the worst they've ever experienced. A Harvard University study involving almost 195,000 men and women over more than eight years found that those who drank just one sugar-sweetened cola per day were 23% more likely to suffer from kidney stones.

DRINK WATER, NOT SUGARY DRINKS, AND LOSE WEIGHT

Consumption of liquid calories has increased in parallel with the obesity epidemic. Researchers from John Hopkins Bloomberg School of Public Health wanted to see how changes in beverage consumption affect body weight in adults. They found that reducing liquid calorie intake, specifically sugar-sweetened beverages, resulted in greater weight loss than reducing solid food intake. Bottom line: Swap sugary drinks for calorie-free drinks like water and lose weight!

LESSON LEARNED

Sugar-sweetened soft drinks are harmful to health and significantly increase your risk of obesity and disease. Don't drink them!

Energy Drinks

GET YOUR ENERGY ELSEWHERE!

THE POPULARITY OF energy drinks—also referred to as "high-concentration caffeine delivery systems"—has skyrocketed over the last decade. They're especially popular with teens and young adults, who have reported drinking as many as five to eight cans in one session. They have enticing names like Red Bull, Monster, Rockstar, Full Throttle, and No Fear. Are these drinks safe? Do they boost energy? Here's what you need to know:

- A typical energy drink, such as Red Bull, contains about 7 teaspoons (35 mL) of sugar and 80 milligrams of caffeine per small can (250 mL/8.3 oz). Some brands in the United States contain as much as 500 milligrams of caffeine in a large serving size. In comparison, a typical can of cola contains about 40 to 50 milligrams of caffeine and a small brewed coffee (8 oz/250 mL) contains about 80 to 175 milligrams of caffeine. Most of the energy-enhancing effects of these drinks are linked to their caffeine content. To date there is limited research supporting the benefits of other ingredients often added to these drinks, such as taurine, glucuronolactone, and guarana.

- Caffeine in moderation is safe and can enhance mood, alertness, exercise performance, and the speed at which a given task is performed. Too much caffeine, however, can cause anxiety, irritability, sleeplessness, and, on occasion, rapid heart rate.

- Excessive energy drink consumption has resulted in some cases of caffeine toxicity and hospitalization. Health Canada recommends that adults limit caffeine to about 400 milligrams daily, and children and teens limit caffeine intake to no more than 2.5 mg/kg body weight. Based on average body weights for children and teens that equates to about:

CHILDREN AGES 4 TO 6	45 mg daily
CHILDREN AGES 7 TO 9	63 mg daily
CHILDREN AGES 10 TO 12	85 mg daily
TEENS (13 PLUS)	110 to 175 mg daily

> FOOD *for* THOUGHT
> "Caffeine-loaded energy drinks have crossed the line from beverages to drugs delivered as tasty syrups."
> **SENIOR EDITORS,** *Canadian Medical Association Journal*

THE BOTTOM LINE If you want caffeine, then get it from coffee or tea instead. Both can be enjoyed with little or no added sugar and they also contain antioxidant-rich plant compounds linked to a lower risk of disease.

Don't underestimate the value of a healthy lifestyle in optimizing energy levels—one that includes lots of nutrient-rich, health-enhancing foods like fruits, vegetables, 100% whole grains, nuts, low-fat dairy, beans, and lean protein. Exercising daily and staying well hydrated is also essential to feeling your best.

ENERGY DRINKS AND YOUR HEART

Researchers from the University of the Pacific in California analyzed data from seven studies to determine the impact of energy drinks on heart health. They found that energy drinks were linked to an increase in blood pressure and a disturbance in the heart's natural rhythm.

ENERGY DRINKS ERODE TOOTH ENAMEL

There has been an alarming increase in the consumption of energy drinks and sports drinks among teens, and it is causing irreversible damage to their teeth. Researchers from Southern Illinois University School of Dentistry looked at acidity levels in 9 different energy drinks and 13 different sports drinks. They found the acidity levels were high enough to erode tooth enamel, the glossy outer layer of the tooth, after just five days of exposure. Teens who consume these drinks are essentially bathing their teeth with acid. Energy drinks were found to be twice as damaging to teeth as sports drinks.

LESSON LEARNED

Energy drinks are often high in sugar and if consumed in excess contain unhealthy amounts of caffeine, especially for young people. Caffeine can boost energy, but should only be consumed within recommended guidelines (see page 42). A healthier way to enjoy caffeine is to drink tea or coffee with little or no sugar added.

Red Meat, Processed Meat, and Colon Cancer

LEAN RED MEAT (beef, pork, lamb) is a valuable source of nutrition, including high-quality protein and vitamin B12, a nutrient not found naturally in plant foods. Red meat contains significant amounts of selenium, niacin, phosphorus, riboflavin, and vitamin B6. Its greatest claim to fame, however, especially for beef, is that it's an exceptional source of highly available (easily absorbed) iron and zinc—two nutrients that many children, women, and seniors don't get enough of. Even mild deficiencies can impair growth, the ability to think and learn, and the ability to defend against infections. By including some red meat in the diet, the needs for iron and zinc are more likely to be met. Too much red meat, however, is linked to a higher risk of disease, including cancer, heart disease, and type 2 diabetes.

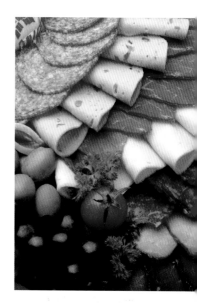

MEAT-EATING HABITS OF OTHER COUNTRIES

The traditional diets of Japan and the Mediterranean region are linked to a long life and low rates of disease. Do these eating plans include meat? Absolutely, but a lot less of it—as much as 4 to 10 times less than Canada and the United States. Meat shows up on their plates, but in small quantities. Don't let meat take the lead role in your diet!

RED MEAT, PROCESSED MEAT, AND CANCER

What's the best reason to reduce your intake of red meat and processed meat? Cancer. To significantly reduce your risk of cancer, especially cancer of the colon, you need to limit red meat and avoid processed meats.

HOW DOES MEAT CAUSE CANCER?

- Red meat contains heme-iron, which in excess can damage the cells that line your colon.
- Heme-iron has the ability to increase the formation of cancer-causing substances in the body called nitrosamines. The nitrites and nitrates added to processed meats can also cause these substances to form.
- Cooking meat at high temperatures and until well-done produces cancer-causing substances called heterocyclic amines (HCAs) and polycyclic aromatic hydrocarbons (PAHs).

- Red meat alters whether specific genes in your body are activated or not. These changes can promote an inflammatory environment, which may promote the development of cancer.

NOT JUST COLON CANCER

Although the greatest link between red meat and cancer is by far colon cancer, meat eating has also been linked to a higher risk of cancers of the stomach, breast, prostate, esophagus, pancreas, lung, liver, endometrium, and bladder.

HOW MUCH MEAT IS SAFE?

The Canadian Cancer Society recommends limiting red meat to 3 servings or fewer per week. One serving is 3 ounces (85 grams or about the size of a deck of cards). They suggest consuming processed meats only on special occasions; for example, ham for a holiday dinner or a hot dog at a sporting event.

MEAT AND CANCER RELAPSE

Based on research from the Dana-Farber Cancer Institute, patients with advanced colon cancer who have undergone surgery and chemotherapy with the goal of cure may have a higher risk of relapsing and dying early if they follow a predominantly "Western" diet of red meat, fatty foods, refined grains, and desserts.

BREAST TISSUE DENSITY, BREAST CANCER, AND MEAT

More and more research suggests that what our teen girls eat while their breast tissue is forming is important in reducing breast cancer risk later in life. If the breast tissue formed is dense, it is strongly associated with an increased risk of breast cancer. In a study from California Polytechnic State University, a high intake of red meat in the teen years was linked to a greater likelihood of dense breast tissue in adulthood.

PROCESSED MEAT AND LUNG HEALTH

Research from Columbia University Medical Center involving over 7,300 men and women with an average age of 65 found that those who consumed processed meats such as bacon, sausage, and cold cuts 14 times or more per month had almost double the risk of developing chronic obstructive pulmonary disease (COPD). Researchers believe that the nitrates added to these products may generate compounds that damage lungs and produce structural changes resembling emphysema. COPD is a major cause of death in the world. Smoking is the greatest risk factor in its development.

SWAP THE MEAT AND PROTECT YOUR HEART

Harvard researchers followed the eating habits of over 84,000 women for 26 years and found that substituting 1 serving of red meat daily for 1 serving of other protein sources was linked to a significantly lower risk of heart disease. Eating 1 serving of nuts instead of meat reduced heart disease risk by 30%, while substituting fish reduced the risk by 24% and substituting poultry reduced it by 19%. In other research from Harvard involving over 21,000 men, red meat was linked to a significantly higher risk of heart failure. Bottom line: Be good to your heart and go easy on the red meat!

RED MEAT AND ARTERY DAMAGE

We know that the saturated fat in red meat can be harmful to our arteries, but that's not all. Researchers from the Cleveland Clinic in Ohio have found that bacteria living in our digestive system convert a compound found in red meat called carnitine into trimethylamine N-oxide, another compound that promotes atherosclerosis or hardening of the arteries. High blood levels of this compound predict a significantly increased risk of heart attack, stroke, and death. In addition, regularly eating a diet high in red meat promotes the growth of bad gut bacteria that convert carnitine into its more dangerous form. Bottom line: Too much red meat is not good for our gut health or our arteries.

MEAT AND WAISTLINE EXPANSION

In a large study by Imperial College London involving over 370,000 men and women from 10 European countries, eating larger quantities of meat was linked to a higher body weight. Over a span of five years, those who ate the most meat (about 9 ounces/250 grams daily) gained about 4.5 pounds (2 kg) in body weight. Imagine what a lifetime of meat eating might cause.

LIMIT MEAT, ESPECIALLY PROCESSED MEAT, TO PREVENT DIABETES

Harvard researchers followed the eating patterns of over 200,000 men and women for 14 to 28 years. Based on this research and a review of other research in the field, they concluded that for every 3.5 ounces (100 g) of red meat you eat daily (a serving size equal to a deck of cards), your risk of type 2 diabetes increases by 19%. Consuming 50 grams of processed meat (equivalent to one hot dog or sausage or two slices of bacon or cold cuts) each day increases your risk by over 50%.

GRILL YOUR MEAT, BUT DON'T GET CANCER

When any kind of meat, poultry, or fish is cooked at high temperatures (frying, grilling, or broiling) and until well-done or charred, cancer-causing compounds called heterocyclic amines (HCAs) and polycyclic aromatic hydrocarbons (PAHs) form. These substances can damage your DNA in ways that make cancer more likely. By following these guidelines you can significantly reduce the formation of these compounds:

- Marinate meat before to cooking (even for just a few minutes) in antioxidant-rich ingredients such as extra virgin olive oil, lemon juice, and herbs and spices. Rosemary and garlic appear to be particularly effective.

- Make hamburgers from scratch and mix herbs, spices, and garlic directly into the patties before cooking.
- Pre-cook meat in the microwave for a few minutes and discard the juice, which contains much of the potentially harmful compounds. Just two minutes of microwaving has been found to reduce HCAS by as much as 90%.
- Cut off all visible fat before grilling. The smoke that rises from the fat that drips onto the coals also produces cancer-causing compounds.
- Cut meat into smaller portions to reduce cooking time.
- Flip meat frequently, every minute or two—this can reduce HCAS by 75% to 90%.

RED ALERT! ANTIBIOTICS, MEAT, AND POULTRY

The routine use of antibiotics in animals leads to the development of antibiotic-resistant bacteria that can be harmful to human health. Meat and poultry purchased at your grocery store can contain high levels of these bacteria. What should you do? Handle raw meat and poultry carefully and cook it properly. Even better, buy meat that comes from animals raised without antibiotics.

VEGETARIANS MUST PLAN WISELY

If you want to follow a vegetarian diet, be prepared to plan your menus wisely. Load up on a wide variety of nutrient-dense foods including fruits, vegetables, whole grains, and low-fat milk products (or milk alternatives such as fortified soy milk). Replace the meat in your diet with plant-based protein sources such as beans, nuts, and nut butters. Don't run short of vitamin B12, a nutrient found naturally only in animal products. Get it from a multivitamin and from consuming foods that are fortified with this nutrient, such as soy milk. A multivitamin will also help you meet your needs for iron and zinc, two nutrients many vegetarians also find challenging to get enough of.

TAKE THE SKIN OFF CHICKEN

When it comes to chicken, whether you eat dark meat or white meat is not so important. White meat is lower in fat and calories. Dark meat contains three to four times more iron and zinc. It's a trade-off. The skin, however, is what you want to leave behind. By removing the skin you cut the calories by as much as 30% and the fat, including the saturated fat, by as much as 50%. That's significant and worth doing!

ROTISSERIE CHICKEN WARNING!

Buying a rotisserie chicken from your local supermarket can be a quick, easy, and tasty meal. Just be sure to remove the skin. Based on research from Kansas State University, the skin of store-bought rotisserie chicken is especially high in cancer-causing compounds. Now you know!

CLEAR THE CONFUSION: PROCESSED MEATS WITH NO NITRATES

Some brands of sliced deli meats are now made with "no added preservatives or nitrates." Are they a better choice? If you are going to buy processed meats, buying meat that is less processed or that contains more natural preservatives is probably a good idea. Understand, however, that researchers are still trying to determine exactly why processed meats are so harmful to health. Until all the answers are in, eating any type of processed meat may still carry some degree of risk.

GOOD ADVICE: HEALTHY MEAT EATING

Here's my meat-eating advice for a healthy eating plan:

- Keep portions sizes small—3 ounces (85 grams or about the size of a deck of cards).
- Go lean and trim all visible fat. "Loin" and "round" cuts are leanest, including beef sirloin and tenderloin (also known as filet mignon) and pork tenderloin. Avoid rib cuts, including prime rib, rib eye, and spareribs: they are the highest in fat. Take the skin off poultry.
- If you buy ground meat, buy "extra lean." Cook and drain off the fat before adding it to spaghetti sauce or other dishes.
- Limit your consumption of red meat to three times per week or less. Choose poultry (skin removed) more often than red meat. Leave plenty of room in your diet for beans (at least four times per week), fatty fish (at least twice a week), and nuts or nut butters (a small handful or serving daily).
- Avoid processed meats or enjoy them just on occasion. They should not be a part of your weekly diet.

LESSON LEARNED

Too much red meat can increase your risk of cancer, especially colon cancer, as well as heart disease and type 2 diabetes. Limit red meat to three times a week or less. It should be lean meat and a serving size no bigger than a deck of cards. Avoid processed meats most of the time. Choose chicken, fish, beans, and nuts more often.

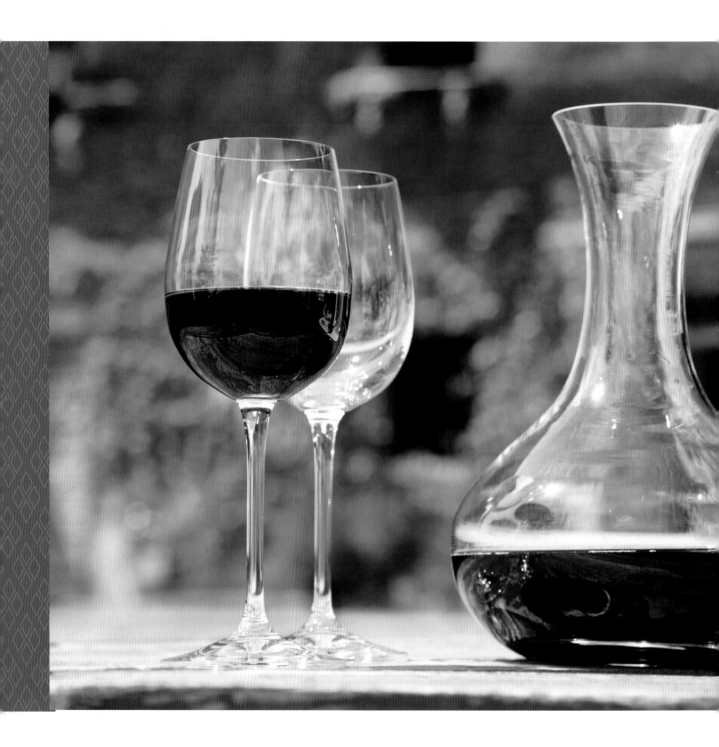

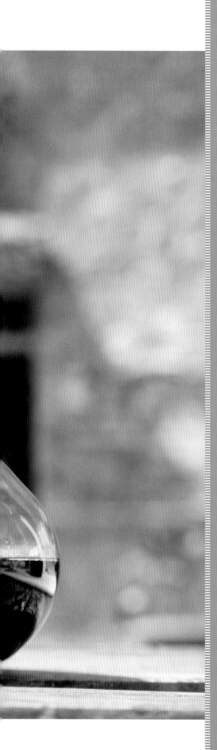

QUESTIONS THAT
NEED ANSWERS

Does a Drink a Day Keep the Doctor Away?

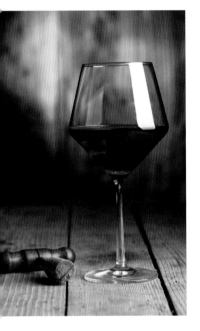

OFTEN WHEN I do a nutrition talk or workshop, someone in the audience will joke with me and say, "just tell me about the red wine and the chocolate!" They don't want to know about the broccoli, the spinach, or the beans. They just want to know about the foods they love, the ones that make them feel good. Alcohol of any kind, however, has been called the "Jekyll and Hyde" of preventive medicine. If you drink a little, it can be good for you. If you drink a lot, it can be bad for you. This is what you need to know about the harmful effects of alcohol:

- A study by the Centre for Addiction and Mental Health in Toronto shows that alcohol is now the third leading cause of disease and injury worldwide, despite the fact that many people in countries around the world abstain from drinking.

- Excess alcohol intake has been linked to more than 200 different diseases and injuries. In excess, alcohol harms the liver, heart, pancreas, and brain. It weakens your immune system, hinders healing, and impairs bone formation. High intakes are linked to liver disease, high blood pressure, stroke, atrial fibrillation (an irregular heartbeat that can lead to stroke), pancreatitis, cancer, depression, suicide, and accidents.

- For those who suffer from alcoholism, alcohol destroys not only the life of the alcoholic, but the lives of family members as well.

THE ALCOHOL–CANCER CONNECTION

Alcohol (ethanol) is classified as a carcinogen by the International Agency for Research on Cancer. It is linked to seven different cancers, including cancers of the breast, colon, larynx (voice box), liver, esophagus, mouth, and throat. The risk increases with the volume of alcohol consumed, especially at an intake of 3 or more drinks a day. Combining smoking with drinking greatly increases the risk. For some cancers, including cancer of the breast, mouth, throat, and esophagus, even light drinking (up to 1 drink a day) can increase risk. That's why organizations such as the American Institute for Cancer Research state that the best protection against cancer is to avoid alcohol entirely. This message is particularly important for those who have a family history of cancer, especially for breast and colon cancer.

ALCOHOL AND CANCER OF THE COLON

The International Agency for Research on Cancer reviewed over 60 studies to determine the link between alcohol and colon cancer. The risk was 20% higher for moderate drinkers (2 to 3 drinks daily) and over 50% higher for heavy drinkers (4 or more drinks daily).

THE GOOD NEWS ABOUT ALCOHOL

Alcohol consumed in moderate amounts has a long history of being good for the heart. The University of Calgary recently reviewed 63 studies to determine just how good it is. Researchers concluded that alcohol in moderation positively affects heart health in three ways:

- It significantly increases your HDL cholesterol—the good kind that carries cholesterol out of the bloodstream and back to the liver for disposal.
- It increases levels of a hormone called adiponectin—a hormone that reduces inflammation or damage to the cells that line blood vessel walls and promotes healthy blood sugar levels.
- It decreases fibrinogen levels, which reduces the stickiness of your blood and, therefore, the risk of a blood clot

causing a heart attack or stroke. The moderate use of alcohol has also been linked to a lower risk of dementia, diabetes, and rheumatoid arthritis.

EXCEPTIONS TO HEART HEALTH BENEFITS

Although alcohol in moderation is good for most people's heart, there are exceptions. Research from McMaster University in Hamilton involving more than 30,000 individuals 55 years or older from 40 countries has found that even moderate drinking is linked to an increased risk of atrial fibrillation (an irregular heartbeat) in older and high-risk heart disease or diabetes patients. An irregular heartbeat is a concern because it significantly increases the risk of stroke. Atrial fibrillation accounts for almost 25% of strokes among elderly people.

ALCOHOL AND YOUR BRAIN

Researchers from Loyola University Chicago reviewed 143 studies to look at the link between alcohol and cognition (the ability to think and learn). These studies overwhelmingly found that moderate drinking either reduced or had no effect on the risk of dementia or cognitive impairment. Overall, light drinking was linked to a 25% lower risk of cognitive decline, and moderate drinking (less than or equal to 2 drinks per day for men and less than or equal to 1 drink per day for women) was linked to about a 30% lower risk. Heavy drinking (more than 3 to 4 drinks per day), however, was linked to an increased risk of

FOOD *for* THOUGHT

"If you do enjoy alcohol, keep your drinking in the moderate range. You don't get any additional heart protection by drinking more. And your risk of cancer—and many other problems—rises dramatically with higher consumption."

HOWARD LEWINE, MD, Chief Medical Editor, Harvard Health Publications

dementia and cognitive impairment. This is consistent with other studies, such as the Health and Retirement Study, which found binge drinking twice a month appeared to more than double the risk of decline in both cognitive function and memory. Bottom line: While a small amount of alcohol may be good for your brain, excess alcohol clearly is not!

IS RED WINE BETTER?

The term "French paradox" was coined in 1992 to describe the relatively low incidence of heart disease in the French population despite a relatively high intake of unhealthy saturated fat. Red wine, it was believed, was the reason why. What we know today is this: All types of alcohol, in moderation, can protect health. It is the ethanol or alcohol itself that provides protection. Red wine, however, appears to provide further protection due to its strong health-protective mix of plant compounds called polyphenols. These compounds are potent antioxidants and promote proper health and function of the blood vessel wall. In the Zutphen Study involving over 1,300 men, long-term wine consumption of, on average, less than half a glass per day was strongly linked to a lower risk of heart disease and a boost in life expectancy of five years.

YOUR PATTERN OF DRINKING MATTERS

Researchers from Toulouse University School of Medicine in France compared the drinking patterns of almost 10,000 middle-age men in France and Northern Ireland over the span of 10 years. The volume of alcohol consumed over a week in both countries was almost the same; however, in Ireland most of the drinking took place over one or two days (weekend drinking) rather than regularly throughout the week. The prevalence of binge drinking was almost 20 times higher in Northern Ireland than in France. The result? The French suffer from considerably less heart disease. They found that men who binge drink (4 to 5 drinks over a short period of time) had nearly twice the risk of heart attack or death from heart disease. Bottom line: If you are going to drink, don't binge.

DRINK IN MODERATION

Moderation is defined by most health organizations as no more than 1 drink a day for women and no more than 2 drinks a day for men. Some researchers, however, feel that just half a drink per day is optimal to minimize risk and still obtain a benefit.

One drink is equal to:

- 12 ounces of beer
- 4 ounces of wine
- 1.5 ounces of 80-proof spirits
- 1 ounce of 100-proof spirits

The healthiest way to consume alcohol is regularly, in small quantities, and with meals. Drinking to intoxication and binge drinking are harmful to health, increase your risk of disease, and cancel out the benefits gained by drinking in moderation. Binge drinking is defined as 4 or more drinks per occasion for women and 5 or more drinks for men.

DON'T FORGET YOUR VEGGIES

If you choose to drink, be sure your diet includes plenty of folate-rich foods. Some research has shown that a folate-rich diet may reduce the risk of cancer associated with alcohol, especially breast and colon cancer. Folate is found in high amounts in dark green and orange vegetables, as well as in beans and lentils.

WHEN YOU DRINK MORE, YOU EAT MORE

We live in a calorie-rich, obesity-promoting environment. Researchers from Uppsala University in Sweden looked at which lifestyle factors make us most vulnerable to excess food intake. The three most prominent lifestyle factors identified were watching television, sleep deprivation, and alcohol intake. All three were found to significantly contribute to excessive eating, with alcohol leading the way. Not only does alcohol contribute calories to your diet, but it also stimulates your appetite, makes food more appealing, and weakens your resolve to make healthy food choices.

THE QUESTION YOU NEED TO ASK

Researchers from Boston Medical Center have found that one simple question (developed by the National Institute on Alcohol Abuse and Alcoholism) helps to identify unhealthy alcohol use: How many times in the past year have you had 5 or more drinks in a day (4 or more drinks if asking a woman)? If your answer is greater than 1, it means your use of alcohol may be unhealthy. Remember, when it comes to alcohol, moderation is the name of the game!

FOOD *for* THOUGHT

"If someone binge drinks even once a month, any health benefits from light to moderate drinking disappear."

J. REHM, MD, Centre for Addiction and Mental Health

LESSON LEARNED

Excess alcohol is harmful to health. It is linked to a higher risk of many diseases, including cancer. Alcohol in moderation is good for your heart. Red wine may provide better protection than other alcoholic beverages due to the antioxidant plant compounds it contains. If you drink, women should consume no more than one drink a day and men no more than two.

Vitamin D

ARE YOU GETTING ENOUGH?

VITAMIN D IS the sunshine vitamin. Your body makes it when sunshine strikes your skin. Getting enough was never a problem for our ancestors. Man evolved naked, in the sun, at the equator. Today, however, many of us live thousands of miles from the equator and spend much of our time indoors. As a result, people are not getting the vitamin D they need. Here's what you need to know about this powerful nutrient.

THE VITAMIN THAT DOES IT ALL

Vitamin D has a tremendous effect on health. It's called the "it" vitamin because there's almost nothing "it" doesn't do. You have receptors for vitamin D throughout your body, including in more than 37 different organs. You have receptors in your brain, muscles, bones, pancreas, cardiovascular system, immune system, and gastrointestinal system, to name a few. When vitamin D attaches to a receptor, it delivers a "message" to the cells in that area. This causes a specific action or response to take place. If there is a lack of vitamin D, these "messages" are not transmitted and your health is compromised. You don't want this to happen.

WHAT HAPPENS WHEN YOU DON'T GET ENOUGH?

Getting enough Vitamin D is important for a strong immune system, strong bones, and strong muscles. It reduces your risk of fractures and falls as you age. It's essential for healthy pregnancies and babies. Lack of vitamin D may increase your risk of some cancers, heart disease, stroke, diabetes (both type 1 and type 2), multiple sclerosis, rheumatoid arthritis, psoriasis, dementia, depression, asthma, and other diseases.

VITAMIN D FOR STRONG BONES AND FEWER FRACTURES

Vitamin D plays a crucial role in the development and maintenance of a healthy skeleton throughout life. Based on a review of 11 studies in the *New England Journal of Medicine* involving more than 31,000 older adults, taking a daily dose of between 800 IU and 2000 IU of vitamin D significantly reduces the risk of most fractures, including hip, wrist, and forearm, in both men and women age

65 and older. No benefit was found in taking vitamin D supplements in doses below 800 IU per day.

VITAMIN D FIGHTS COLON CANCER

Living at higher latitudes with less sun exposure is associated with an increased risk of a variety of cancers and an increased risk of dying from them. Vitamin D appears to reduce cancer risk by slowing the progression of cells from the pre-malignant to malignant states. The strongest evidence is for colon cancer. A review of 18 studies by researchers from Shanghai found that a higher intake of vitamin D, along with higher blood levels, was linked to a significantly lower risk of colon cancer.

HAPPINESS AND VITAMIN D

Emerging research suggests that if you suffer from depression or have a history of depression, you may want to make sure your needs for vitamin D are being met. Researchers from St. Joseph's Hospital in Hamilton, Ontario, reviewed 14 studies involving over 31,000 participants and found a significantly higher risk of depression in people with low levels of vitamin D.

LOW VITAMIN D MEANS HIGHER RISK OF DEATH

In a 10-year study from the German Cancer Research Center involving over 5,000 men and women over the age of 50, lack of vitamin D was linked to an increased risk of death overall, including a higher risk of death from heart disease, cancer, and respiratory disease.

HOW MUCH DO YOU NEED?

The Institute of Medicine states that infants (birth to 12 months old) should get 400 IU of vitamin D (a supplement is required if breast-fed). Children (age 1 and up) and adults should aim for 600 IU of vitamin D a day. You need 800 IU if you are over the age of 70. These numbers, however, remain quite controversial; some researchers and organizations believe they should be higher. The Canadian Cancer Society, for example, suggests talking to your doctor about taking 1,000 IU of vitamin D during the fall and winter months. Other researchers say getting closer to 2,000 IU each day is ideal. More research in this area is required.

THE SUNSHINE VITAMIN

Just a short time in the sun—with exposed skin, without sunscreen, for 5 to 10 minutes between 10 a.m. and 3 p.m. two to three times per week—can meet the need for vitamin D. However, in countries that are above 40° north latitude (Northern United States and all of Canada) or below 40° south latitude (Southern South America and Southern New Zealand), the sun is not strong enough to make vitamin D in the winter months. In addition, if you have dark skin, are obese, or over the age of 70, your body may not be as efficient at making vitamin D. In these cases, a supplement is probably a wise idea.

VITAMIN D: FOOD OR SUPPLEMENT?

Very few foods are naturally good sources of vitamin D, with the exception of higher-fat fish like salmon (3 ounces/85 grams contains about 300 IU). In many countries, including Canada and the United States, certain foods, such as milk and margarine, are fortified with vitamin D but at fairly low levels. For example, a glass of milk contains 100 IU of vitamin D. To make sure your needs for vitamin D are met, most people need to take a supplement. I take 1,000 IU of vitamin D daily (in addition to the vitamin D that I get in my multivitamin and in my food). Children age 9 and above and all adults should limit their intake of vitamin D (from food and supplements) to no more than 4,000 IU each day. The suggested upper limit for younger children is between 1,000 to 3,000 IU, depending on age (specific dosage guidelines are available through the Institute of Medicine). Ongoing research over the next decade should help to clarify the optimal requirement for this important nutrient.

CAN YOU GET TOO MUCH?

The most common side effect of having too much vitamin D is high levels of calcium in the blood, which can lead to kidney stones and deposits of calcium in organs and soft tissues. For most people this only happens when taking very high doses of vitamin D supplements combined with calcium supplements. I recommend people get all or most of their calcium from food and only take calcium supplements to top up if they need to (see guidelines for calcium intake on page 85). Keep your intake of vitamin D within the recommended upper limit (no more than 4,000 IU each day for adults).

GET TESTED

Everyone should have a blood test to check their vitamin D level once a year. You want to achieve a blood level of at least 20 to 30 ng/mL (50 to 75 nmol/L). The optimal blood level for the prevention of disease is still being determined.

LESSON LEARNED

Vitamin D is absolutely critical to good health. It lowers your risk of a long list of diseases. Children and adults need at least 600 IU daily, and 800 IU as you get older. Some researchers believe getting 1,000 to 2,000 IU (especially in the winter months) may be ideal. Most people need to take a supplement in order to meet their needs for this powerful health-protecting nutrient.

Is Taking a Multivitamin Good Sense or Nonsense?

SHOULD YOU TAKE a vitamin and mineral supplement? This is a very important question to ask. The right supplement can provide strong health protection and prolong life. The wrong supplement can cause significant harm, even death. Here's what you need to know.

THERE IS NO MAGIC BULLET

No pill can replace the magic of a healthy, balanced diet. Fruits, vegetables, whole grains, beans, and nuts contain an intricate mix of vitamins, minerals, antioxidants, and fibre, along with literally hundreds of beneficial plant compounds—all of which interact in an incredible dance of health protection and disease prevention that can't be manufactured in a pill. Your primary focus should always be on good, wholesome, healthy food!

DEFICIENCY HAS CONSEQUENCES

What if you're not optimizing your nutritional intake through diet? What if you're not consuming the recommended amounts of fruits, vegetables, grains, dairy, and protein? Research says very few people are. A recent study by the NDP Group in the United States looked at how often the average consumer meets at least 70% of the recommended dietary guidelines. The results were dismal. Success was achieved only 2% of the time or seven days out of the whole year—bad news! Researchers are now finding that even mild deficiencies of some nutrients can damage cells over time and may increase the risk of cancer and heart disease as well as compromise the health of the immune system and brain. While there is no question that people need to put far more effort into eating a nutritious and balanced diet, we can't ignore the fact that for many people a supplement may be beneficial, too.

TOO MUCH OF A GOOD THING

Taking a supplement can be a very risky business. The American Heart Association says "almost any nutrient can be potentially toxic if consumed in large quantities over a long time." Taking high amounts of individual nutrients, especially in isolation, appears to be especially dangerous. High doses of vitamin A have been linked to birth defects and weaker bones. Extra beta-carotene, selenium, folic acid, and vitamin E have all been associated with an increased risk of some cancers. Your risk of cataracts may go up with too

> FOOD *for* THOUGHT
> "Almost any nutrient can be potentially toxic if consumed in large quantities over a long time."
> **AMERICAN HEART ASSOCIATION**

much vitamin C or E. Calcium in excess has been linked to kidney stones as well as heart attacks and strokes. Too much iron is particularly toxic; it can damage organs and cells and increase your risk of many chronic diseases. Bottom line: Supplements must be approached with caution. They are not to be played with—not if you care about your health.

A MULTI MAKES SENSE

Other than vitamin D and fish oil (see pages 80 and 38), the only supplement I recommend at this time is a multivitamin (and possibly calcium if you are unable to meet calcium needs through food and only enough to make up for dietary shortfalls; see page 85). I believe a multivitamin is the safest way to make sure nutritional needs are covered without causing unnecessary harm. Some researchers suggest taking a multivitamin every *other* day just to minimize the risk of excess nutrients of any kind. It's a viable option. It is also recommended that if you take a multivitamin, you should minimize your intake of heavily fortified foods. Some cereals, drinks, and energy bars, for example, contain significant amounts of added vitamins and minerals. You don't want to get more nutrients than you need in this way.

WHAT TO LOOK FOR IN A MULTI

With so many kinds of multivitamins to choose from, how do you choose wisely? *Consumer Reports* tested 21 different brands and found that all but one met label claims for key nutrients, none contained worrisome levels of contaminants, and most passed the dissolution test (which shows they dissolve properly in your body). Store brands or generic brands, like Costco's Kirkland Signature, tested just as well as the national brands but sold at much lower prices. I think as long as you stick with well-known, bigger brands (including store brands) you should be fine.

Buying a multivitamin designed for your gender and age, such as silver formulas for the senior years, is also good practice. Women, for example, need very different amounts of iron prior to menopause, during pregnancy, and after menopause. Too much or too little iron can be harmful to health. You can always compare your multivitamin to the recommended nutrient intakes for your age as set out by the Institute of Medicine (fnic.nal.usda.gov/dietary-guidance/dietary-reference-intakes/dri-tables). Try to choose a formula that is close to what you really need.

POPULATIONS AT RISK

Some people need a multivitamin more than others. Vegetarians often don't get enough nutrients from food, including vitamin B12 and iron. Vitamin B12 is also an issue for people age 50 and above, as they may no longer have enough stomach acid to extract it from food. In general, the older we get, the more challenging it is to meet overall nutrient needs. Women who are trying to get pregnant (or those who could get pregnant) should take a multivitamin to ensure they are getting adequate folic acid. When taken in the first few weeks of the pregnancy, often before a woman even knows she's pregnant, folic acid plays a significant role in the prevention of neural tube defects (defects in the brain and spinal cord of the child).

WHAT'S MISSING?

The US Dietary Guidelines Advisory Committee published a list of seven nutrients that most people don't get enough of in their diets:

- calcium
- fibre
- folate
- iron
- potassium
- vitamin B12
- vitamin D

Other potential shortfall nutrients include vitamin A, vitamin C, vitamin E, vitamin K, choline, and magnesium.

VITAMIN C AND THE COMMON COLD

Researchers from the University of Helsinki in Finland reviewed 72 studies to determine the effect of vitamin C supplements (200 milligrams and higher) on the incidence, severity, and duration of the common cold. Their conclusion: Taking vitamin C on a daily basis is not justified for most people. It does not reduce the risk of the common cold. They did find, however, that vitamin C was helpful in preventing colds in those who participate in really intense physical activity, such as marathon runners. In addition, they found that adults and kids who take vitamin C as soon as they catch a cold may shorten its duration by a day or two.

THE BOTTOM LINE The recommended intake for vitamin C is 75 milligrams daily for women and 90 milligrams for men. Smokers need an additional 35 milligrams. These needs can easily be met through diet, especially if your diet includes 1 to 2 daily servings of any of the following vitamin C-rich fruits or vegetables: citrus fruits or juices, papaya, bell peppers, strawberries, broccoli, kiwi, cantaloupe, or dark leafy greens. Taking high doses of vitamin C (about 1,000 mg) on a daily basis has been linked to a higher risk of kidney stones and cataracts.

LESSON LEARNED

No pill will ever replace food for optimal health and the prevention of disease. Most people, however, do not meet nutrient needs through diet. A multivitamin is the safest way to supplement the diet and to make sure all of your nutrient needs are met.

Does Milk Fit into a Healthy Diet?

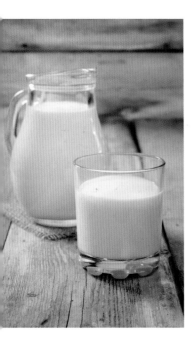

DO YOU CONSUME 2 to 3 servings of milk products a day (or milk alternatives such as fortified soy milk)? Most children, teens, and adults do not. Many people underestimate the value of milk, while others believe it may even be harmful to health. What do I think? Milk fits into a healthy diet and is worthy of our attention. Here's why.

MILK DELIVERS FAR MORE THAN JUST CALCIUM

Our bodies need nutrient-dense foods, today more than ever! Few foods contain as much nutrition as a glass of milk. It's a powerhouse of protein, vitamins, and minerals. Every single glass you drink significantly increases your overall nutritional intake. Every single glass you don't drink significantly compromises your overall nutritional intake. This is true for many nutrients including protein, calcium, potassium, magnesium, vitamin D, vitamin B12, riboflavin, vitamin A, phosphorus, and zinc. That's a lot of nutrition you don't want to miss out on!

MILK AND BONE HEALTH

Bone is a living tissue that is always changing. Bone growth occurs primarily in childhood. Girls usually experience a "bone growth spurt" between the ages of 11 to 14 and boys between the ages of 13 to 17. By about age 20 our bones have stopped growing and our job is to maintain the bones we have. Calcium is recognized as the most critical nutrient for the achievement of optimal peak bone mass. Without adequate calcium, it is not possible either to build or maintain a fully normal skeleton. Milk is an exceptional source of calcium, as well as an important source of other bone health nutrients, including protein, magnesium, phosphorus, and potassium.

OSTEOPOROSIS: THE DISEASE OF FRAGILE OR BRITTLE BONES

Osteoporosis Canada states that one in three women and one in five men will have an osteoporotic fracture during their lifetime. This is a disease that can severely reduce one's quality of life, causing chronic pain, depression, reduced mobility, and loss of independence. About one-fifth of older adults who fracture a hip will die within six months; of the survivors, half will not be able to walk without assistance, and half will need full-time nursing care. The best way to prevent osteoporosis is to build and maintain a healthy bone mass, starting in childhood. An active lifestyle is also important.

CALCIUM FROM OTHER SOURCES

What about getting your calcium from other calcium-containing foods like broccoli, kale, bok choy, almonds, and beans? These foods can contribute significant amounts of calcium to your diet, especially if you eat a lot of them. Without milk products as part of the mix, however, most adults and kids don't meet recommended calcium intakes (not to mention the fact that milk contributes so many other nutrients to your diet as well). Fortified soy milk is the only true milk alternative as it provides all the key nutrients found in milk, including calcium.

WHAT ABOUT ALMOND, RICE, OR COCONUT MILK?

Almond, rice, and coconut milk all contain less calcium than cow's milk or fortified soy milk, unless additional calcium has been added. They also contain significantly less protein and potassium (a nutrient most people don't get nearly enough of) and they may or may not be fortified with vitamin B_{12} and vitamin D. If you prefer to use one of these milk alternatives, almond milk is the most nutritious option. Just be sure to choose a brand that is fortified with extra calcium, vitamin B_{12} and vitamin D. Also make sure your diet is rich in potassium (including lots of dark green and orange fruits and vegetables) and that you consume at least two to three protein-rich foods daily, such as lean meat, fish, chicken, beans (legumes), nuts or nut butters.

CALCIUM FROM A PILL?

Taking a calcium supplement may be good for your bones, but it may also be harmful to your heart. Researchers from the University of Auckland in New Zealand reviewed 15 studies involving over 20,000 participants and found that taking calcium supplements (500 milligrams or more daily) was linked to about a 30% greater risk of having a heart attack. Ongoing research will tell us more. The bottom line: Do your best to get your calcium from food. Get 2 to 3 servings of milk products a day. Each serving provides about 300 milligrams of calcium. Eating an overall healthy, well-balanced diet will deliver another 300 milligrams, especially if you make an effort to consume foods that are calcium-rich. Only take a supplement to top up any shortfalls you can't get through diet. The recommended calcium intake for women ages 19 through 50, and men up to age 70, is 1,000 milligrams daily. Women over 50 and both men and women 71 and older require 1,200 milligrams of calcium each day.

BEYOND BONE HEALTH

In many countries around the world, people don't consume the recommended daily number of milk products. Researchers

FOOD *for* THOUGHT
"There are few true replacements for the nutrient package you find in one glass of fat-free or low-fat milk."
KEITH AYOOB, MD, RD,
Pediatric Nutrition Expert,
Albert Einstein College of
Medicine

from the University of South Australia reviewed the scientific literature to determine how a low intake of milk affects healthcare costs and the overall burden of disease. They found strong evidence to support a higher risk of obesity, stroke, heart disease, type 2 diabetes, high blood pressure, and osteoporosis in those who don't consume enough milk products. The healthcare cost attributable to low milk intake was estimated to be about $2 billion a year, which is comparable to the total amount spent on public health in Australia. Other research also links a low consumption of milk products to a higher risk of tooth decay, periodontal disease, kidney stones, and gout. Bottom line: Not consuming enough milk is costly to individuals and countries.

THE TRUTH ABOUT LACTOSE INTOLERANCE

Lactose is a sugar naturally found in milk and milk products. An enzyme called "lactase" is needed for your body to break down or digest this sugar. If you don't have enough of this enzyme, you may experience symptoms like bloating, gas, stomach cramps, and diarrhea when you consume certain milk products. This condition is more common in people of African American, Hispanic, and Asian descent. Many people, however, mistakenly believe that they suffer from lactose intolerance and remove milk products from their diet without undergoing proper testing. Even if you are properly diagnosed, most people can tolerate ½ to 1 cup (125 to 250 mL) of milk

at one sitting with minimal symptoms, especially when milk is consumed with other foods. In addition, most yogurt and hard cheeses (like cheddar, Swiss, Parmesan, and mozzarella) can be included in the diet as they contain very little lactose. Consuming lactose-free milk and taking lactase supplements (tablets or drops) are other options. Perhaps most important is that good research shows the gut can be reconditioned. By consuming small servings of milk throughout the day and slowly increasing the amount over two to three weeks, you alter gut bacteria and the ability to digest lactose improves significantly. Taking certain kinds of probiotics can help with this process. Organizations, such as the American Academy of Pediatrics, state that "the elimination of milk products to treat lactose intolerance should be considered a last resort."

HOW MUCH MILK?

Most kids and adults need 2 to 3 servings of milk products a day, along with a healthy, well-balanced diet.

One serving is equal to:

- 1 cup (250 mL) of milk or fortified soy milk
- ¾ to 1 cup (185 to 250 mL) of yogurt
- 1.5 ounces (50 g) cheese or ⅓ cup (80 mL) of shredded cheese

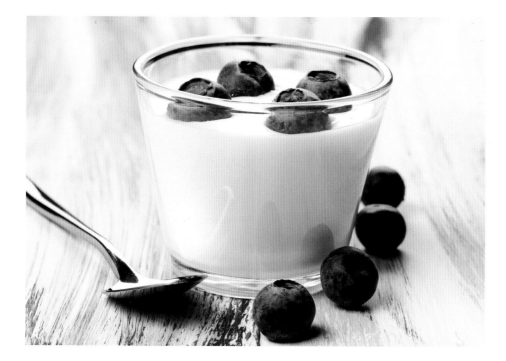

WHICH MILK
PRODUCTS ARE BEST?

I give first place to fat-free milk (skim milk) or 1% milk, and low-fat yogurt (those with added probiotics also qualify). These choices are low in fat and have the highest nutritional value per calorie.

Second place belongs to flavoured yogurts. These generally contain less nutrition and as much as 3 to 6 teaspoons (15 to 30 mL) of added sugar per 1 cup (250 mL). Look for brands that are low-fat (no more than 3 grams of fat per serving or 2% MF or less), contain less sugar, and are highest in calcium. Those with added probiotics are also a good choice. Greek yogurt, while significantly higher in protein, is often lower in much-needed calcium (some brands more so than others) as well as potassium. It's a trade-off. If

you like Greek yogurt, include other milk products in your daily diet, too.

Cheese ranks third place. Although most of us love cheese (myself included!), it's a concentrated source of fat, calories, and sodium. Enjoy it in smaller quantities and choose lighter varieties when possible (look for brands with less than 20% MF). Most soft cheeses, such as feta, brie, Camembert, and goat cheese, contain significantly less calcium than hard cheeses, such as cheddar, Swiss, mozzarella, and Parmesan. Ricotta cheese contains about four to five times more calcium and significantly less salt than cottage cheese. Cream cheese contains very little calcium. Low-fat frozen yogurt and, to a lesser extent, light ice cream can also contribute calcium and other nutrients to your diet. Enjoy them as an occasional treat and limit serving size to about ½ cup (125 mL).

MORE WAYS TO UP YOUR INTAKE

Enjoy a latte or cappuccino made with low-fat milk. If oatmeal is a part of your morning breakfast, make it with low-fat milk rather than water. Rather than buying pre-sweetened yogurt, buy low-fat plain and add your own fruit (along with a dash of maple syrup or honey, if needed). Make fruit or veggie dips with yogurt. Add milk or yogurt to smoothies rather than juice.

DOES CHOCOLATE MILK FIT INTO A HEALTHY DIET?

Milk naturally contains about 3 teaspoons (15 mL) of milk sugar per cup (250 mL). Chocolate milk contains all of the wonderful nutrients you find in plain milk, but with 3 teaspoons (15 mL) of added sugar—about 50 extra calories.

Can chocolate milk fit into a healthy diet? Strong research shows that children and teens drink significantly more milk when it's flavoured. This means they get significantly more nutrition, including more calcium at a time when their bones and bodies really need it. It's also a time when many other drinks, including soft drinks, are competing for their attention. Many organizations, including the American Dietetic Association, the American Academy of Pediatrics, and the American Heart Association state that the benefits of drinking low-fat flavoured milk outweigh the harm of the added sugar.

If you decide to include chocolate milk in your diet or your family's diet, look for brands that contain less added sugar. When you make chocolate milk at home, add just 1 teaspoon (5 mL) of syrup, rather than the 3 teaspoons (15 mL) suggested by most companies. Last but not least, if you're looking for a good sports recovery drink for you or your kids (only needed after exercising an hour or more at a moderate to high intensity), chocolate milk provides a good balance of fluids, carbohydrates, electrolytes, and protein.

LESSON LEARNED

Milk products, especially low-fat milk and plain yogurt, are a very concentrated source of nutrition. They support good health, including bone health. Overall nutrient needs, including calcium, are compromised if milk products are not consumed. Even people with lactose intolerance can learn to fit milk products into their diet. Aim for 2 to 3 servings a day.

How Much Water Should We Really Drink?

THERE ARE MANY things in life you can live without. Water is not one of them. Just a few days of deprivation and the consequences can be lethal. This isn't surprising when you consider that the majority of your body—about 60%—is water. That's a lot of water, but then again, every cell in your body needs it. It's essential for digestion, delivering nutrients, carrying away waste, regulating your body temperature, cushioning joints, and a whole lot more! Your body loses water every day, primarily through sweat and urine, and that water must be replaced.

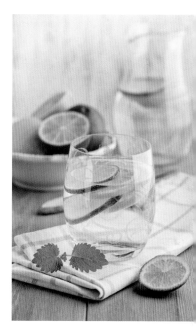

DRINK WHEN YOU'RE THIRSTY

How much water do you really need? Guidelines from the Institute of Medicine state that for the vast majority of healthy people "the combination of thirst and usual drinking behaviour, especially the consumption of fluids with meals, is sufficient to maintain normal hydration." Purposefully drinking more is recommended when you're active (especially for sustained, vigorous activity) or when you're exposed to heat (like when you are outdoors on a hot summer's day). Additional guidelines come from the European Food Safety Authority based on a recent and extensive scientific review. They define an adequate water intake for most women as 6½ cups (1.6 L) daily and for most men as 8 cups (2 L) daily. This amount includes beverages of all kinds, not just water. Coffee, tea, milk, juice, and other beverages count toward your daily quota. This guideline assumes that you live in a moderate climate, are moderately active, and that an additional 20% of your overall need for water will be met through food. Most fruits and vegetables, for example, are at least 80% water and significantly contribute to your daily intake.

THE IMPACT OF DEHYDRATION

Dark yellow urine is a sign of dehydration. Even mild dehydration can drain your energy and make you feel tired. Since water makes up about 75% of your brain, not getting enough can lead to headaches and affect your ability to think, learn, and concentrate. There is also a link between dehydration and a greater risk of high blood sugar, gallstones, and constipation. Keeping yourself hydrated is important!

YOUR KIDNEYS NEED WATER

If you care about your kidneys (and you should!), getting enough water or other fluids has to be a priority. Your kidneys are absolutely essential to good health. They filter waste out of your blood and dispose of that waste in your urine. Strong evidence says that not drinking enough water significantly increases your risk of kidney stones, which can be extremely painful, and compromises the long-term health of your kidneys, including your risk of chronic kidney disease. A lack of water may also raise your risk of urinary tract infections.

DRINK BETTER, THINK BETTER

Researchers from the University of Connecticut studied the impact of mild dehydration on cognitive function in a group of 26 men and 25 women. The level of dehydration was typical of what most adults might experience one or more times during the course of a week. In both men and women, dehydration had an adverse effect on mood as well as on the ability to concentrate. It also resulted in fatigue, declines in short-term memory, and headaches. Bottom line: To feel well and think well, you must hydrate well.

OLDER ADULTS
DON'T DRINK ENOUGH

As we get older the water content of our body decreases along with our ability to detect thirst. Dehydration is more common, more serious, and one of the top 10 causes of hospitalization for seniors. It

can result in medication toxicity, kidney failure, seizures, and a significantly higher risk of falls as well as death. Raising water awareness in older adults, as well as families and caregivers, is important. Water or other fluids should be consumed and encouraged regularly throughout the day and with meals.

SPORTS NUTRITION

The amount of water lost through sweat when exercising varies greatly depending on the person, the type of activity, and the duration. Dehydration can lead to muscle fatigue, loss of coordination, inability to regulate body temperature, and decreased athletic performance. It's best to drink extra water before, during, and after exercise. A sports drink with added carbohydrates and electrolytes may be necessary if exercise is more vigorous and lasts an hour or more.

WATER GETS TOP SPOT

A panel of experts from the University of North Carolina reviewed 146 studies to come up with the Beverage Guidance System. The goal was to rank beverages from the best to the worst based on their calorie and nutrient content, as well as their ability to protect or harm health. When their review was complete, guess which beverage was number one on their list, the one they want you to drink most often? If you guessed water, you're right. Water is calorie-free yet vital for good health. At the bottom of their list, not surprisingly, were sugar-sweetened beverages such as soft drinks. Are your beverage choices healthy? Does water get top spot in your day?

WHICH WATER IS BEST?

For most people, tap water is a fine choice. Mineral water can contribute significant amounts of much-needed calcium and magnesium to your diet, but choose brands that are lower in sodium. Bottled water, in most cases, is no better for you, is generally more harmful to the environment, and may not contain added fluoride, which contributes to good dental health. Vitamin water is not recommended: Many brands are high in sugar. The best way to get your vitamins is through a healthy diet, along with a multivitamin that contains a balanced amount of all nutrients. Coconut water is a natural and relatively low-calorie way to hydrate yourself; it contains about 35 to 45 calories per 1 cup (250 mL) and is very rich in potassium—a nutrient most of us don't get nearly enough of and one that is really important for healthy blood pressure. Choose brands that contain no added sugar and are lower in sodium.

DRINK UP!

An easy way to up your water intake is to carry a reusable water bottle with you at all times. To make water more appealing, especially at home or in the office, jazz it up with slices of lemon, lime, orange, or other fresh fruit, such as berries or watermelon. You can also add sliced cucumber, thinly sliced gingerroot, and fresh herbs, including fresh mint, rosemary, thyme, or basil. Allow these infusions to steep in the fridge for 2 to 24 hours depending on the strength of the flavour you prefer. Both coffee and tea are also healthy ways to get more water and antioxidants into your day (as long as you watch your caffeine intake and drink them without added cream and sugar).

LESSON LEARNED

You can't live without water. Most women need to drink about 6½ cups (1.6 L) a day; most men need 8 cups (2 L) a day. All beverages, including coffee, tea, milk, and juice, count toward your daily quota. A low water intake can affect your energy, your ability to think and learn, and your overall health, especially the health of the kidneys.

Is It Time to Put Eggs Back on the Menu?

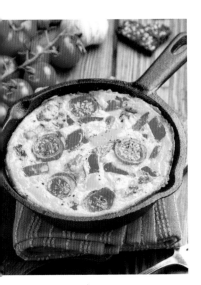

IS IT OKAY to eat eggs even though they contain cholesterol? A solid body of research shows that for most people, cholesterol in food has a much smaller effect on the levels of cholesterol in your blood because your body compensates by manufacturing less cholesterol itself. Other factors, such as the type of fats you eat, have a far greater effect. To keep your blood cholesterol levels healthy, focus on replacing saturated fats with healthy fats—those found in vegetable oils, fish oils, and nuts—and avoid trans fats completely. Maintaining a healthy body weight, exercising regularly, and eating lots of cholesterol-friendly foods like beans, fruits, vegetables, and high-fibre whole grains is also important. The bottom line: Eggs can fit into a healthy diet for most people, with a few exceptions. Read on to find out more.

THE HARVARD EGG STUDY

Research from Harvard involving more than 117,000 participants found no link between eating eggs and the risk of heart disease or stroke in normal healthy men and women, even at the highest intake of one egg per day. They did, however, find that people with diabetes who ate more than one egg per day had as much as double the risk of heart disease. Harvard researchers recommend that people with diabetes limit their egg intake to three eggs per week. Both the American and Canadian Diabetes Association recommend the same.

BIG NUTRITION IN A SMALL PACKAGE

Eggs contain a whole lot of nutrition in one small package. They're an excellent source of high-quality protein and a solid source of 14 essential nutrients, including vitamin A, vitamin B12, vitamin D, vitamin E, riboflavin, folate, iron, selenium, and choline. They're rich in lutein and zeaxanthin, which are potent antioxidants essential for eye health that may reduce the risk of macular degeneration and cataracts. Plus they're low in saturated fat and contain only about 75 calories per large egg. They're also affordable, taste great, and easily fit into a busy lifestyle.

EGGS AND CHOLINE

Eggs are the single most concentrated source of choline, a nutrient that many people don't get enough of. Choline is needed for the normal functioning of all cells, including brain cells. It enhances brain development in babies, improves memory after birth, and reduces the risk of having a baby with birth defects. It's also needed for normal liver function—lack of choline is linked to a higher risk of fatty liver and liver damage. Other sources of choline include lean beef, pork, salmon, shrimp, navy beans, soybeans, wheat germ, flaxseeds, and pistachios.

PROCEED WITH CAUTION: CHOLESTEROL HYPER-RESPONDERS

While the cholesterol found in foods like eggs doesn't appear to have a significant impact on blood cholesterol levels in most people, about 15% to 30% of people are considered "hyper-responders," which means their blood cholesterol levels increase significantly when they eat cholesterol-rich foods. People who are overweight, sedentary, and suffer from diabetes appear to be most likely to fall into this category.

PROCEED WITH CAUTION: THE EGGS–DIABETES LINK

Researchers from the University of North Carolina reviewed 16 studies involving over 90,000 men and women to determine the impact of eggs on heart health and diabetes. Consuming one egg a day was not linked to a higher risk of heart disease or stroke in healthy people; however, it was linked to a 42% higher risk of type 2 diabetes. In addition, daily egg eaters who suffered from type 2 diabetes increased their risk of heart disease by almost 70%. Bottom line: Eggs are not risk-free. We still have more to learn, including a better understanding of the egg–diabetes link. Animal studies suggest that high cholesterol intakes impair the pancreas's ability to release insulin, the hormone that removes excess sugar from the bloodstream.

COUNTING YOUR EGGS

What is a safe amount of eggs to consume based on what we know today? Some experts say eating one egg a day is okay for healthy people. Based on the possible eggs–diabetes link, however, I believe we should proceed with caution and consume no more than one egg three to four times per week. This guideline is especially important for people who are overweight and sedentary or suffer from heart disease or diabetes.

DON'T DISCARD THE YOLK

Some people discard the egg yolk because it contains the cholesterol. The yolk, however, also contains most of the vitamins and minerals and almost half of the protein. Enjoy the whole egg, but don't consume more than one whole egg on any given day.

FOOD *for* THOUGHT

"Dietary cholesterol has been greatly oversold as a health concern, in part because it has a small effect on blood cholesterol levels. Some of the foods that contain high cholesterol, such as eggs, have many other healthy components."

WALTER WILLETT, MD, Harvard University

"It is more important to emphasize diets including fibre-rich, nutrient-dense, plant-based foods than focus on restricting foods high in cholesterol or saturated fat."

JOSEPH CARLSON, RD, Professor, Michigan State University

SKIP THE BACON AND SAUSAGES

The healthiest way to enjoy your egg is with other healthy foods. Make a one-egg omelette loaded with onions, mushrooms, green or red peppers, diced tomatoes, and fresh herbs. Round out your meal with a piece of 100% whole-grain toast and perhaps a glass of low-fat milk. I'm getting hungry! How about you?

BUY OMEGA-3 EGGS

These designer eggs are produced by chickens fed special diets that include foods such as flaxseeds or algae. They are significantly higher in omega-3 fats and vitamin E. Some chickens are also fed marigolds to produce eggs that are higher in lutein, a nutrient important for eye health.

FOOD *for* THOUGHT

"For those at risk of cardiovascular disease or who have type 2 diabetes, eating too many eggs 'could be as bad as cigarette smoking.'"

DAVID JENKINS, MD,
Nutrition Professor
and Researcher,
University of Toronto

LESSON LEARNED

Eggs are a nutrient-dense food, an excellent source of protein, and a rich source of health-protective nutrients like lutein, zeaxanthin, and choline. Daily consumption, however, may increase the risk of diabetes. The risk of heart disease may also increase in those who are overweight, sedentary, and suffer from diabetes. Limit eggs to about three or four per week (especially important for those in the high-risk group).

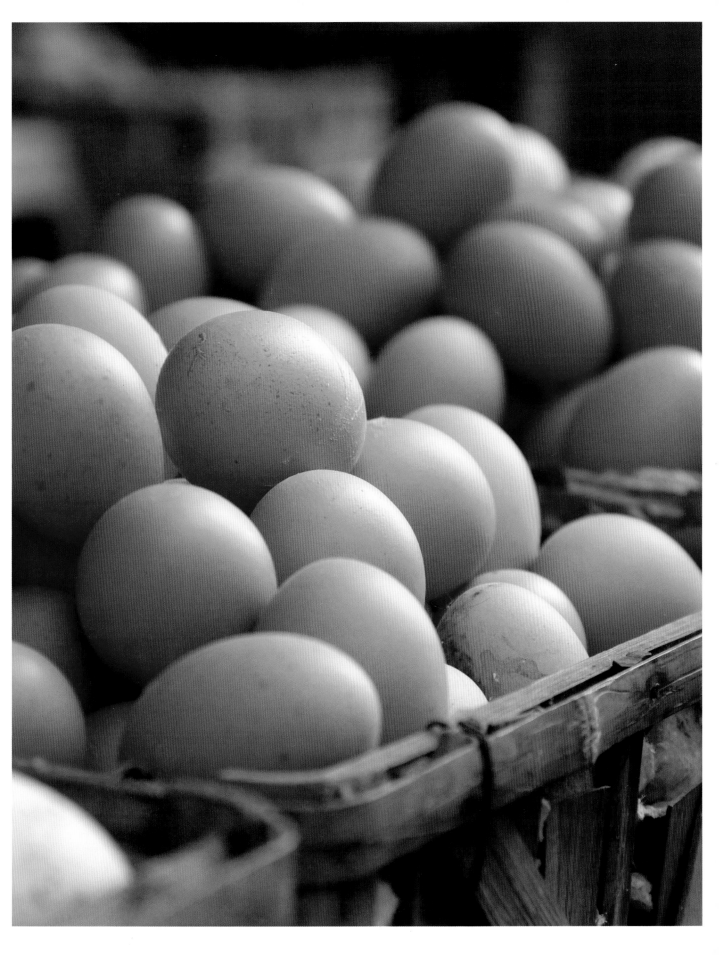

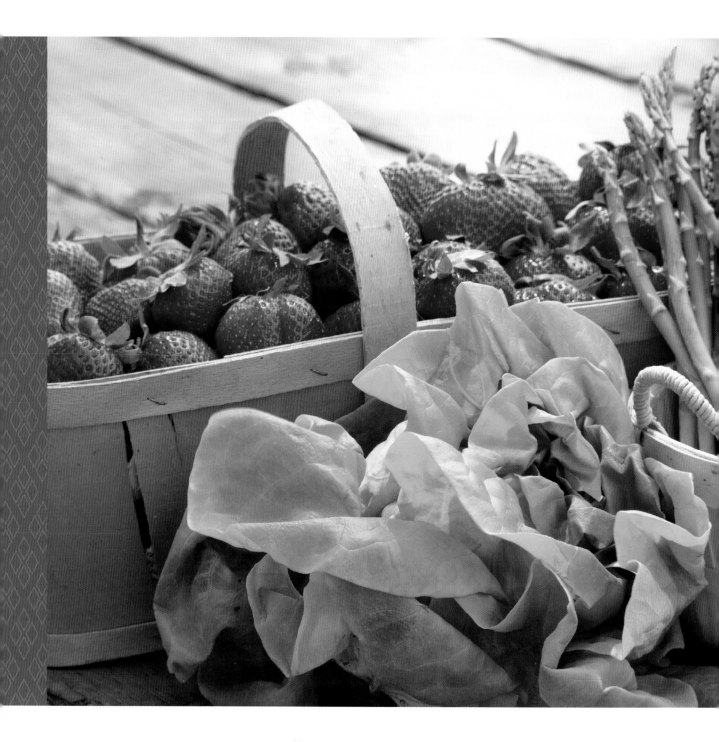

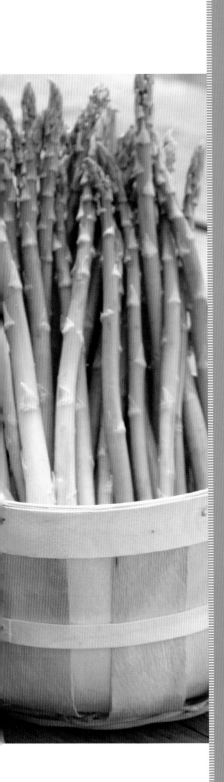

MAKING SENSE
OF FOOD MYTHS AND
MISUNDERSTANDINGS

Ten Things You Should Know About Fruits and Vegetables

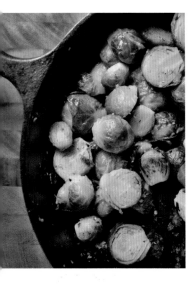

OU KNOW THAT fruits and vegetables are good for you and you should eat lots of them. You know they're loaded with health-protective vitamins, minerals, fibre, antioxidants, and other good stuff. What you may not know, however, is just how good they are. In addition, you may be confused about which ones are best, whether to buy organic, and how to get your kids to eat them. Read on for 10 things I want you to know about fruits and vegetables.

1. Colour Protects Health

Fruits and vegetables with the most vibrant colours—the dark greens; the bright oranges and reds; the brilliant blues, blacks, and purples—contain the most nutrients and valuable plant compounds, including powerhouse nutrients like magnesium, potassium, folate, beta-carotene, and vitamin C, along with health-protective, antioxidant-rich plant compounds that fight disease. Here's a list of colourful fruits and vegetables you should reach for often:

DARK GREEN artichokes, asparagus, broccoli, bok choy, Brussels sprouts, dark leafy greens (spinach, kale, watercress, etc.), green peppers, kiwi, peas

ORANGE apricots, cantaloupe, carrots, oranges and other citrus fruits, mangoes, papaya, pumpkin, squash, sweet potatoes

RED apples, beets, cherries, cranberries, grapefruit (red or pink), guava, pomegranate, raspberries, red cabbage, red peppers, strawberries, tomatoes, watermelon

BLUE/BLACK/PURPLE blackberries, blueberries, dates, eggplant, figs, grapes, plums (fresh and dried/prunes), raisins

2. Fruits and Vegetables Are Good for Bones

Fruits and vegetables don't just reduce your risk of heart disease and cancer. They also build strong bones. Researchers from Tufts University found that eating the equivalent of about 9 servings of fruits and vegetables a day helps to keep bones strong. By increasing the alkali content of the diet, fruits and vegetables help neutralize acids that cause bone to break down or "turn over" as we age. Other studies, like the Framingham Heart Study, also link a lifelong intake of fruits and vegetables to strong bones in the later years.

3. Fruits and Vegetables Slim Your Waistline

Research at Pennsylvania State University involving 71 obese women found that a diet rich in fruits and vegetables was more effective for weight loss than a low-fat eating plan. Fruits and vegetables, especially those high in water and fibre such as broccoli, carrots, spinach, apples, berries, kiwi, and citrus fruits, provide fewer calories per bite than most other foods. They fill people up and satisfy hunger, but don't come with a high cost to the waistline. They are the best weight loss secret there is.

4. Fruits and Vegetables Lower Blood Pressure

U.S. News & World Report evaluated and ranked 29 diets with input from a panel of health experts. To be top-rated, a diet had to be relatively easy to follow, nutritious, safe, and effective for weight loss, as well as for preventing and managing diabetes and heart disease. The competition was fierce, but the top spot (best diet overall) was taken by the DASH diet (Dietary Approaches to Stop Hypertension). DASH promotes eating 8 to 10 servings of fruits and vegetables a day, along with low-fat dairy, whole grains, nuts, and beans (legumes). Known for its ability to lower blood pressure quickly—often in just 14 days!—this diet is so effective that it can prevent the need for blood

pressure–lowering medication. Research also links this fruit-and-vegetable-rich diet to a lower risk of obesity, cancer, heart failure, and kidney stones. Is there anything fruits and vegetables don't do?

5. Fruits and Vegetables Make You Feel Good!

Researchers from the University of Warwick studied the eating habits of 80,000 people in Britain. Those who ate at least 7 servings of fruits and vegetables a day were found to be the happiest and had the best mental health. The researchers stated that "the statistical power of fruits and vegetables was a surprise." Researchers from the University of Otago in New Zealand found the same to be true when looking at the eating habits of almost 300 young adults over a period of 21 days. Participants reported feeling calmer, happier, and more energetic on the days they ate 7 to 8 servings of fruits and vegetables. Healthy foods and happy moods really do go together!

6. Should Vegetables Be Eaten Raw or Cooked?

Eat a wide variety of both raw and cooked vegetables. Some nutrients, like vitamin C and folate, are easily lost during cooking. Other nutrients, like beta-carotene and lycopene, become more available to the body. When you do cook vegetables, steam, microwave, or stir-fry them. Use as little water as possible and short cooking times. Your cooked vegetables should be tender-crisp. Use medium, not high, heat

FOOD *for* THOUGHT
"Currently, there is no convincing evidence that shows a difference between organic and conventionally grown foods related to cancer risk. The advantages of including more vegetables and fruits in your diet strongly outweigh any potential risks from pesticides."
THE AMERICAN INSTITUTE OF CANCER RESEARCH

when stir-frying. Most importantly, don't boil your veggies (unless you're having soup). You lose too much nutrition and disease-fighting power in the water.

7. Fruit Juice Can Harm Health

A glass of fruit or vegetable juice often provides a powerful hit of antioxidants and nutrition. That's a good thing. Too much juice, however, can be bad for health. In a study involving over 100,000 men and women, Harvard researchers found a link between increasing fruit juice intake and diabetes. Fruit juice contains a lot of sugar (about 6 to 8 teaspoons/30 to 40 mL per cup/250 mL) and calories (about 120 to 150 calories per cup/250 mL). Limit yourself to no more than half a cup (125 mL) to 1 cup (250 mL) of 100% fruit juice daily and drink it with meals. Both orange and pink grapefruit juice are good choices and especially rich in vitamin C, potassium, and folate. Black, purple, or blue juices (pomegranate juice in particular!) get top marks for the powerful, disease-fighting antioxidants they provide. With vegetable juice, limits are not as important if you stick to lower-sodium options. Tomato juice is rich in lycopene, a health-protective nutrient that's not found in many other foods.

8. Organic Is Good, but Not Mandatory

The term "organic" is used for plant foods grown without pesticides. More research is required to truly understand the potential benefits and risks. For vulnerable groups, including children, pregnant women, and breast-feeding women, buying organic produce is a reasonable decision, especially when buying produce that is more likely to contain pesticide residues (the Environmental Working Group provides an updated list of the worst offenders at www.ewg.org). For everyone else, if you can afford organic fruits and vegetables, it's worth it to buy them: they may be safer, higher in antioxidants, and better for the environment. They often taste better. Buying them, however, is not mandatory. What is mandatory? Eating 7 to 10 servings of fruits and vegetables day in and day out!

9. Genetically Modified Fruits and Vegetables Are Okay

Foods that are genetically modified (the DNA or genetics of part of the plant is changed in some way) often result in increased crop production, lower food costs, and increased farmer safety as fewer pesticides are required. Are they safe for us to eat? David Zilberman, a University of California at Berkeley agricultural and environmental economist, says, "The benefits of genetically modified crops greatly outweigh the health risks, which so far remain theoretical." The American Association for the Advancement of Science, the World Health Organization, and the exceptionally vigilant European Union all agree that genetically modified foods are just as safe as other foods. The bottom line: While some researchers suggest expanded safety testing is required, the

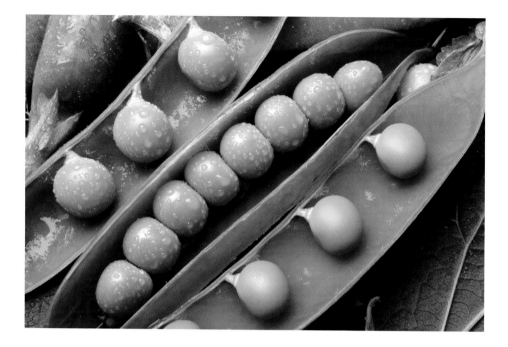

vast majority of research on genetically modified foods (including fruits and vegetables) says that they are safe to eat.

10. Getting Kids to Eat Their Veggies

A review of 60 studies by Loughborough University in the United Kingdom concluded that the most powerful influence in promoting vegetable consumption among kids was "seeing their parents eat and enjoy them." This principle holds true for most healthy foods. "Availability in the home" and "encouraging but not pressuring kids to eat their veggies" was also important. If a particular vegetable is initially rejected by your kids (or other family members!), keep serving it. The more times a vegetable shows up on the plate, the more likely it is to eventually be accepted.

LESSON LEARNED

Fruits and vegetables are all-star health protectors. Enjoy them raw or cooked. Limit fruit juice and choose low-sodium vegetable juice. Organic produce can be a better choice, especially for children, pregnant women, and breast-feeding women. If you want your kids to eat their vegetables, eat and enjoy them yourself.

Snacking Should Be
Your Friend, Not Your Enemy

IS SNACKING HEALTHY or harmful? It depends. For many people, unhealthy snack choices are harming health and causing waistlines to expand. For those who choose wisely, however, the benefits of good snacking are immense. This is what you need to know.

DOES SNACKING IMPROVE YOUR NUTRITIONAL INTAKE?

Non-stop snacking has become a national pastime for many people. Consuming at least three snacks a day is the norm, and as much as one-third of calories are coming from snacks. Regular snacking is linked to a higher intake of some healthy foods (for example, fruit). However, many children, teens, and adults are getting more sodium, sugar, unhealthy fats, and calories than they need because of poor snack choices, including salty snacks, cookies, candy, and desserts. As much as 50% of snack calories are coming from beverages, including fruit drinks, sports drinks, soft drinks, and specialty coffee drinks. Bottom line: Most people are choosing snacks that don't provide good nutrition. Some researchers believe that trying to promote healthy snacking is not enough and that we need to put far more emphasis on getting people to stop snacking on the stuff that isn't good for them.

SNACKING AND YOUR WAISTLINE

Healthy snacking can stave off hunger, keep your appetite in check, and prevent overeating at meals. Most people, however, succumb to the unhealthy snack choices that surround them at home, work, or school. These unhealthy choices don't fill up or satisfy people because they're lacking in fibre, protein, and good nutrition. People also snack mindlessly, not tuning in to what, how much, or how often they're eating. They snack in front of the television and computer, often when lonely or bored. What's the result? Obesity and an increased risk of disease. If you want a healthy body, you have to be a healthy snacker.

ARE YOUR HABITS HEALTHY?

Researchers from Utrecht University in the Netherlands wanted to determine what factors were most strongly linked to unhealthy snacking. They found that the most important predictor, outperforming all other variables, was whether or not it was a habit to choose unhealthy snacks.

In other words, if you are a person who frequently and automatically reaches for unhealthy snacks, without really thinking about it, you are also the person most likely to make unhealthy snack choices. It sounds so simple. What does this mean for you? Habits are fine, as long as they are good habits. Get in the habit of frequently and automatically reaching for snacks that provide good nutrition. That's how you become a healthy snacker.

DOES TIMING MATTER?

Does it matter if you snack in the morning or at night? Researchers from Health Care Food Research Laboratories in Tokyo measured the health impact of eating a snack in the morning (10 a.m.) compared with the evening (11 p.m.) over a period of 13 days. Eleven healthy women, average age 23, participated in this trial. Compared with daytime snacking, nighttime snacking significantly decreased fat oxidation (less stored fat was broken down to produce energy) and increased total and LDL (bad) cholesterol levels. Researchers concluded that eating at night changes fat metabolism and increases the risk of obesity. What do I think? By the time nighttime rolls around, most people have had more than enough calories. Do most of your snacking during the day!

LOCATION, LOCATION, LOCATION!

You've heard that location matters when it comes to real estate. Well, it really matters when it comes to food, too. Research from Utrecht University in the Netherlands says if you want to keep your snacking under control, move your snacks farther away. A bowl of snacks was randomly placed either 8 inches (20 cm), 28 inches (70 cm), or 55 inches (140 cm) away from study participants. The closer the snack, the more likely it was to be consumed. The bottom line: Keep healthy snacks (fruits and vegetables) close by and in sight. Move less-healthy snacks out of sight and out of reach. Better yet, don't have them around at all. Make it easy to reach for the good stuff and super easy to avoid those foods that do not serve you well.

TURN OFF THE TUBE!

Researchers from Deakin University in Australia reviewed 53 studies involving children, teens, and adults to see how sedentary behaviour affects food intake. The news was not good. Television viewing in particular was strongly linked to an increased consumption of unhealthy snacks, drinks, and fast food and a decreased consumption of fruits and vegetables. Watching television exposes people to commercials for unhealthy food and also distracts them, making them less aware of the amount of food they're actually eating. In some cases, people consume a substantial portion of their daily calories in front of the television. Don't make TV time unhealthy snack time.

POTATO CHIPS REALLY ARE ADDICTIVE!

We tend to eat some foods, such as potato chips, more for pleasure than for hunger.

Now we know why: Researchers from Friedrich-Alexander University in Germany compared the brain activity of rats fed standard chow with those fed potato chips. They found that eating potato chips activated the addiction and reward centres in the brain. What does this mean for you? If you find certain unhealthy foods difficult to stop eating once you start, your best choice may be not to start eating them at all.

SMALL SNACKS SATISFY

Researchers from Cornell University measured how hungry or satisfied people felt 15 minutes after eating a small snack (under 200 calories) or a larger snack (over 300 calories). The results showed that smaller portions are capable of providing the same feeling of satisfaction as larger ones. Make all your snack choices smaller, especially the not-so-healthy ones!

GO FOR A WALK INSTEAD

People often snack on unhealthy foods at work to deal with the stress or boredom of the job. Research from the University of Exeter in England found that a 15-minute walk cut snacking on candy at work in half. Taking a short break away from your desk appears to keep your mind off food and reduces your tendency to snack mindlessly. Exercise is known to have significant benefits for mood, energy levels, and managing addictions. Get up and get walking!

LESSON LEARNED

Snacking is only as healthy as the snacks you choose. Most people are snacking too often and choosing unhealthy, processed snacks that significantly increase the risk of obesity and disease. For optimal health, developing healthy snack habits must be a priority.

Definition of a Healthy Snack

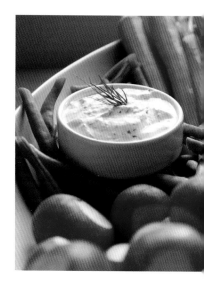

IF HEALTHY SNACKING is good for health, what does a healthy snack look like? Here are three factors to consider: A healthy snack should provide significant nutritional value. It shouldn't be too high in calories, sugar, sodium, or unhealthy fats. It should complement your meals and fill in the dietary shortfalls. Here are more specific snack guidelines:

1. Plan your snacks. This is critical to good snacking. Keep your house stocked with healthy snacks and always pack snacks-to-go before heading out the door.

2. Keep the calorie content of each snack within the 100 to 200 calorie range. If meals are larger, snacks should be smaller and vice versa.

3. Choose snacks that are more natural and less processed. For example, eat a whole apple with the skin on rather than having apple juice or applesauce.

4. Choose foods that provide significant nutritional value, including fruits, vegetables, 100% whole grains (breads, crackers, cereal, popcorn), nuts, seeds, nut butters, milk (or soy milk), yogurt, cheese (in moderation), and beans (edamame or hummus).

5. Snack on foods that you normally don't get enough of each day. For example, most people don't eat the recommended daily servings of fruits and vegetables. Make a deal with yourself: You won't reach for another type of snack until you eat a fruit or vegetable first.

6. Include a source of protein in your snack, such as milk, yogurt, cheese, nuts, seeds, nut butters, or beans. This will give your snack more staying power.

7. Avoid snacks that appear healthy but are not. Here are some tips to follow:

   • Avoid fruit roll-up or gummy bear–like snacks. Stick to dried fruit (in small amounts) or better yet, plain, whole fruit.

- Stay away from hazelnut or other nut-based spreads that list "sugar" as the first ingredient on the label. Real nut butter lists "nuts" as the first ingredient.

- Most 100-calorie snack packs have little nutritional value.

- Just because cookies are low in fat or organic doesn't mean they're good for you.

- Many granola bars are more like candy bars. Look for ones that are lower in sugar and unhealthy fats and higher in fibre (4 to 5 grams per bar). They should contain primarily healthy ingredients like 100% whole grains, nuts, seeds, and dried fruit.

FOOD *for* THOUGHT
"Snacking isn't 'bad' if you do it in moderation and make healthy choices."
THE AMERICAN HEART ASSOCIATION

10 HEALTHY SNACK IDEAS

1. A piece of fruit with a small handful of nuts. Have an apple with some walnuts, a banana with some almonds, or a clementine with some peanuts.

2. Cut-up veggies and dip. Serve carrot sticks, red pepper strips, or broccoli florets along with hummus or a black bean or Greek yogurt dip.

3. A homemade smoothie made with milk or yogurt and fresh fruit or veggies.

4. A piece of 100% whole-grain toast or half a whole-grain bagel with peanut or almond butter.

5. Plain, low-fat yogurt mixed with fresh fruit. Add low-fat granola for a homemade parfait.

6. A handful of trail mix made with nuts, dried fruit, and whole-grain cereal.

7. A few slices of light cheddar cheese served with whole-grain crackers.

8. A small bowl of whole-grain cereal or oatmeal with low-fat milk.

9. A small bean salad, edamame, or roasted chickpeas (see page 221).

10. A latte or hot cocoa made with low-fat milk or soy milk.

LESSON LEARNED

Choose snacks that are less processed, more nutritious and not too high in calories, salt, sugar, or unhealthy fats. Foods such as whole fruits and vegetables, low-fat milk or yogurt, nuts, 100% whole grains, beans, and bean dips all qualify.

Drink Coffee, Live Longer

ALL COFFEE LOVERS rejoice (I know there are a lot of you out there!). Coffee is more healthful than harmful. While tea is still my beverage of choice for health, more and more research says that coffee can do a body good. It can lower your risk of disease and even help you live longer. Here is the latest and greatest news on a beverage that has many adoring fans.

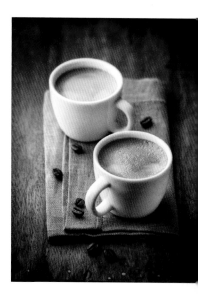

RICH IN ANTIOXIDANTS

Coffee, like tea, comes from a plant. For those who drink it regularly, it is a major source of antioxidants in the diet (both regular and decaf). The antioxidant compounds in coffee, including caffeic, ferulic, and p-coumaric acids, along with the caffeine, protect health. They've been shown to prevent damage to cells caused by free radicals, decrease inflammation, and improve sensitivity to insulin (you need less insulin to move sugar out of your blood and into your cells).

THE GOOD NEWS ABOUT COFFEE

Some of the strongest research support for coffee and disease reduction is for type 2 diabetes. Each cup you drink provides further protection. Drinking 3 to 4 cups per day is linked to a 25% lower risk of type 2 diabetes. Regular coffee drinkers are also at a lower risk for dementia (including Alzheimer's), Parkinson's, stroke, gallstones, gout, and depression. Early research even says coffee may lower the risk of some cancers, including cancer of the liver, colon, mouth, throat, endometrium, and prostate.

YOUR LIVER LIKES COFFEE

Your liver is a very important organ in your body. It's been called your body's "inspection station." Its main job is to filter and clean the blood coming from your digestive tract before allowing that blood to pass to the rest of your body. Regular, moderate coffee consumption is linked to a lower risk of many types of liver disease, including fibrosis (scar tissue that builds up in the liver) and cirrhosis (the result of a long-term buildup of scar tissue within the liver) as well as liver cancer.

WHAT ABOUT YOUR HEART?

Researchers from Sun Yat-sen University in China reviewed 21 studies and concluded that over the long term, coffee does not increase the risk of heart disease. This conclusion held true for those who were light, moderate, heavy, and very heavy coffee drinkers. Note, however, that drinking unfiltered coffee, such as Turkish, French press, and Scandinavian boiled coffee, has been linked to an increase in LDL (bad) cholesterol and triglycerides. When you filter coffee, you remove a substance (cafestol) that appears to have cholesterol-raising properties. Espresso has less cafestol than boiled or French press coffee, but more than paper-filtered coffee.

SHOULD YOU DRINK DECAF?

While drinking decaf coffee is always an option, drinking coffee with caffeine appears to provide better overall health protection. For example, cancer studies have shown that caffeine helps inhibit tumour progression. With dementia, caffeine helps block inflammation in the brain. Caffeine provides other benefits, too. In moderation it improves alertness and concentration. It helps with jet lag, keeps you attentive while driving, and if you do shift work, it improves your ability to work well. It's also linked to improved sports performance and a reduction in muscular pain.

IS IT ADDICTIVE?

Contrary to what many believe, caffeine is not considered a drug of dependence. However, regular coffee drinkers who give up their coffee-drinking habit suddenly do experience withdrawal symptoms, including headaches, difficulty concentrating, and drowsiness. This can be avoided by cutting back more gradually.

HOW MUCH CAFFEINE IS TOO MUCH?

Health Canada recommends limiting your intake of caffeine from all sources to 400 milligrams a day. One small cup of coffee (8 oz/250 mL) or a shot of espresso contains anywhere from about 80 to 175 milligrams of caffeine (depending on the type of bean, processing, and preparation). Drinking between about 2 to 4 small cups of coffee a day keeps you within the recommended limit for caffeine (you can have more if it's decaf). Remember, however, that this guideline is based on an 8-ounce (250 mL) coffee. If, for example, you order the "grande" coffee (16 oz/500 mL) from Starbucks, you need to count it as 2 cups.

WHAT HAPPENS IF YOU EXCEED YOUR LIMIT FOR CAFFEINE?

Consuming more than the recommended daily limit for caffeine may cause problems such as restlessness, anxiety, and irritability, especially in those who are more sensitive to caffeine (some people metabolize caffeine more slowly than others). It can interfere with sleep, making it more difficult to fall asleep, stay asleep, and sleep deeply. Consuming most of your caffeine in the morning and early afternoon is generally best. In excess, caffeine may also cause abnormal heart rhythms in those who are predisposed.

FOOD *for* THOUGHT
"I think the evidence that coffee is a healthy beverage is pretty substantial now; it seems to be beneficial across the board."
ERIC RIMM, MD,
Professor, Harvard
School of Public Health

During pregnancy and while breastfeeding, women should limit caffeine. Health Canada recommends a limit of 300 milligrams of caffeine a day during pregnancy (some organizations advise 200 milligrams or less).

THE CAFFEINE CONTENT VARIES

How much caffeine does that cup of coffee or espresso really contain? It's hard to know. The amount of caffeine from one cup to the next varies greatly depending on the amount of coffee used, the type of bean, and the preparation method. In one study by the University of Glasgow, the caffeine content of espresso coffee from 20 different shops was measured. They found that levels of caffeine differed as much as sixfold. One coffee shop's coffee contained as much as 322 milligrams of caffeine. This means you might be taking in a lot more caffeine than you realize. Women who are pregnant or breast-feeding need to be especially aware of this fact.

DOUBLE CREAM AND SUGAR

Coffee contains next to nothing in terms of calories. What you add to your coffee, however, can really add up, especially if you enjoy several cups a day. Most of us already get too much sugar in our diet, and cream is not only rich in calories (60 calories in 2 tablespoons/30 mL of light cream), but also very high in fat—the kind your heart doesn't like! Drink coffee black or with milk, and no sugar. Sugar substitutes used in small amounts are an option. A latte or cappuccino made with low-fat milk is a good choice. Most importantly, watch out for specialty coffees and iced coffees from your local coffee shop. A medium-size Vanilla Frappuccino from Starbucks contains 430 calories, 14 grams of fat (9 of which are the not-good-for-your-heart kind), and 17 teaspoons (85 mL) of sugar. That's insane! That's not a coffee—it's a decadent dessert! The nutritional information for most coffee products is now available online, including the caffeine content. Check the numbers before you damage your health and your waistline.

LESSON LEARNED

Coffee is more healthful than harmful and is linked to a lower risk of type 2 diabetes, liver disease, and more. Both the antioxidants and the caffeine in coffee can protect health. For most people, 2 to 4 small cups of caffeinated coffee a day is a safe limit (depending on your caffeine intake from other sources). If you'd like more, drink decaf, which also protects health.

The Health of Your Gut Determines the Health of Your Body

YOU HAVE LITERALLY trillions of bacteria inhabiting your body, most of which live along the entire length of your gastrointestinal tract. In fact, a healthy human intestinal tract hosts 10 times as many bacteria as there are cells in the human body. You are a living factory of bacteria. Is this bad? No, not if the bacteria that reside in your body are mostly the "good" or "friendly" kind. If, however, your body is overpopulated with "bad" or "harmful" bacteria, your health may be severely compromised. Here is what you need to know.

HEROES FOR YOUR HEALTH

The "good" bacteria that live in your body are enormously important to your health. There is almost nothing they can't do! These bacteria are crucial to a healthy immune system—about 70% of your immune system resides in your gut! They are your first and primary defence against harmful bacteria, toxins, and allergy-causing proteins. They communicate intimately with the immune cells that are concentrated in your small intestine. In the colon, they produce antimicrobial agents that provide protection against harmful bacteria and viruses as well as compounds that fight cancer. They create barriers that stop toxins from entering your body. These good or friendly bacteria are also essential for the digestion of food, helping you get energy and process vitamins, minerals, and antioxidants. They help your body absorb calcium, make vitamin K, and efficiently handle fats and sugars.

WHEN GOOD BACTERIA ARE IN SHORT SUPPLY

What happens if you don't have enough of the "good" bacteria working hard to keep you healthy? You may increase your risk of infection, including the common cold, bronchitis, pneumonia, and the flu. Your risk of many different types of disease may increase, including inflammatory bowel diseases, skin diseases (like dermatitis, psoriasis, and eczema), rheumatoid arthritis, and cancer of the colon. You may be more likely to suffer from diarrhea, constipation, gas, inflammation, lactose intolerance, stomach ulcers, and food allergies. Your chance of having a heart attack or stroke may increase, as well as your risk of developing diabetes. Lack of good bacteria can even affect your ability to maintain a healthy body weight, your energy level, and your overall well-being. A healthy gut has a huge impact on your health!

THE OPTIMAL GUT ENVIRONMENT

How do you keep your gut healthy and the "good" bacteria thriving? What you eat on a daily basis has a huge impact on gut health. A diet made up of lots of processed and refined foods and high in sugar and unhealthy fats is extremely detrimental to gut health. In contrast, a diet rich in whole fruits and vegetables (with the skin on), 100% whole grains, beans, nuts, and seeds contributes significantly to the health of your gastrointestinal tract. As for antibiotics, take them only if you need to. Antibiotics not only kill harmful bacteria, but healthy bacteria as well.

WHAT ARE PREBIOTICS?

In simple terms, prebiotics are food for "good" bacteria. They help the good bacteria in your gut grow and thrive. For a food or ingredient to qualify as a prebiotic, it must contain substances that are resistant to absorption and digestion, such as fibre. When prebiotic substances reach the colon they are fermented and provide food for the good bacteria to grow. Consuming a diet that is very high in fibre (more beans, please!) and loaded with plant foods (whole grains, nuts, fruits, and vegetables) is important. Specific food ingredients, including inulin and resistant starch, have also been identified as prebiotic.

WHAT ARE PROBIOTICS?

Probiotics are live bacteria that when consumed in adequate amounts are beneficial to your health. Fermented foods (for example, yogurt, buttermilk, kefir, sauerkraut, miso, tempeh) are a source of live bacteria. The amount of live bacteria they contain, however, is quite variable. Probiotic supplements and food items like yogurt that contain "added live bacterial cultures" have very large, standard doses of bacteria (billions of healthy bacteria, usually lactobacillus or bifida bacteria) and, therefore, are more likely to have a significant impact on gut health.

Should you take a probiotic supplement or eat foods that contain added probiotics? Eating a healthy, high-fibre, plant-based diet is one of the most important things you can do for gut health. Eating foods or taking a supplement with added live bacteria, however, can provide additional protection. We still have much to learn. Prebiotic and probiotic research is still in its infancy. Scientists are still trying to determine which strains of bacteria (as many as 1,000 different strains live in your gut) are most important to good health. Different types or strains of bacteria are linked to different health benefits. For example, one strain may be beneficial for constipation, while another may reduce your risk of infection. If you choose to consume a food item with added probiotics (dairy products are considered a great carrier for probiotics) or if you take a probiotic supplement, choose a well-known brand. Brands like Dannon,

Yoplait, Bio-K Plus, and Jamieson have good research support behind the probiotic products they produce.

IF YOU TAKE ANTIBIOTICS, TAKE PROBIOTICS, TOO!

Researchers from RAND Health in California reviewed 63 studies involving more than 11,000 participants and found that taking probiotics was linked to a 42% lower risk of developing the diarrhea that is a common side effect of taking antibiotics. Further research will tell us which strains are most effective for the prevention of this kind of diarrhea.

GOOD GUT HEALTH IS GOOD FOR HEART HEALTH

In animal research from the Medical College of Wisconsin, it was found that the types of bacteria in the intestines might be used to predict a person's likelihood of having a heart attack and that manipulating these organisms may help to reduce heart attack risk. The researchers believe that their discovery is a revolutionary milestone in the prevention and treatment of heart disease. Bottom line: A healthy gut and a healthy heart go hand in hand.

PROTECT YOURSELF FROM HARMFUL TOXINS

Heavy metals such as lead, mercury, and arsenic frequently contaminate food and water. The "good" or "friendly" bacteria that reside along your gastrointestinal tract are capable of degrading pesticides as well as binding and detoxifying toxic chemicals. About 40% to 60% of metals ingested by humans do not breach the intestinal barrier, and host bacteria play an important role in preventing entry. One more reason to say thank you to your healthy gut bacteria!

LESSON LEARNED

The "good" or "friendly" bacteria that live along your gastrointestinal tract have a tremendous impact on your health. They are crucial to a healthy immune system and play an incredible role in the prevention of disease. A high-fibre, plant-based diet helps support a healthy gut and provides food for the bacteria that live there. Foods or supplements with added live bacteria (probiotics) can provide additional protection.

The Truth about Gluten-Free Diets

WILL FOLLOWING A gluten-free diet help you to lose weight, feel better, and feel more energetic? Celebrities are endorsing it. Gluten-free products now line store shelves. Restaurants are serving gluten-free options. Is this a fad or does the gluten-free craze make good sense? Here's what you really need to know:

- When people who have celiac disease eat gluten—a protein found in wheat, barley, and rye—it triggers an abnormal immune response that damages the lining of the small intestine. This damage reduces the intestine's ability to absorb nutrients from food and can be harmful to health. Symptoms include anemia, chronic diarrhea, weight loss, fatigue, cramps, and bloating. Diagnosis is done with blood tests and a biopsy of the small intestine. The only treatment available at this time is to follow a gluten-free diet.

- Health Canada estimates about 1 out of every 100 to 200 people worldwide suffers from celiac disease. It can occur at any age. If someone in your immediate family has it, you have a 10% to 20% higher risk of developing it. Children who are breast-fed may be less likely to develop it, especially if foods that contain gluten are introduced gradually in small amounts at age five to six months and breast-feeding is continued for at least one month after gluten is introduced.

- The number of people who suffer from celiac disease has been increasing worldwide. The cause of the increase is still not understood. Some researchers, such as Dr. Alessio Fasano from the Center for Celiac Research and Treatment, believe that environmental factors such as an infection, taking antibiotics, or a change in diet can alter gut bacteria and make people more susceptible to the disease. What can you do to promote a healthy gut environment? Eat a diet that contains lots of whole unprocessed foods, including fruits, vegetables, beans, nuts, and 100% whole grains. Probiotics, such as those added to yogurt, may also be beneficial.

> FOOD *for* THOUGHT
>
> "It is well possible that many individuals are on a gluten-free diet for no sound medical reasons."
>
> **ALESSIO FASANO, MD, Center for Celiac Research**

- Some people do not have celiac disease but display a sensitivity to gluten. This involves a different type of immune reaction in which there is inflammation but no damage to the intestine. Symptoms can be similar to celiac disease. Total elimination of gluten from the diet may not be necessary; however, eating fewer foods that contain gluten and eating them in smaller quantities may be helpful. There is no official diagnosis for gluten sensitivity. Removing gluten from the diet and then gradually re-introducing it while keeping a food diary may be the best way to monitor symptoms.

- Should you follow a gluten-free diet if you don't have to? Will it give you more energy, help you lose weight, or prevent disease? You should only follow this diet if you suffer from celiac disease or demonstrate a definite sensitivity to gluten or wheat. Books that promote a gluten-free diet for everyone, such as *Wheat Belly*, are not well supported by scientific fact. People who omit gluten from their diets are more likely to miss out on important nutrients such as iron, B vitamins, and fibre. These diets may also cause a reduction in the number of good or healthy bacteria that live along the gastrointestinal tract, which are so important to good health. Most importantly, there is strong research support for eating a wide variety of 100% whole grains, including those that contain gluten, especially when these grains are consumed in the least processed state. Their consumption is linked to a lower risk of many diseases, including heart disease, diabetes, and cancer. Enjoying a wide variety of grains is a much more enjoyable way to eat too.

- If you must follow a gluten-free diet, understand that many gluten-free products are made with refined grains like corn or potato starch that are low in fibre and lacking in the nutrients and beneficial plant compounds found in whole grains. They're often unfortified as well, which means they are not good sources of B vitamins or iron. It is important to make gluten-free choices that are still 100% whole grain, such as quinoa, buckwheat, teff, sorghum, amaranth, millet, brown rice, and wild rice. Bean-based flours also offer good nutrition (soy, chickpea, lentil). Oats are generally allowed as long as they are pure and uncontaminated. Many of the oats in North America are processed near or with grains that contain gluten.

LESSON LEARNED

People with celiac disease cannot eat grains that contain gluten, including wheat, barley, and rye, because it damages their small intestine and their health. Those who suffer from a sensitivity to gluten may have to limit their intake as well. For others, there is no need to limit or omit gluten from the diet and, ultimately, doing so may be more harmful to health than beneficial.

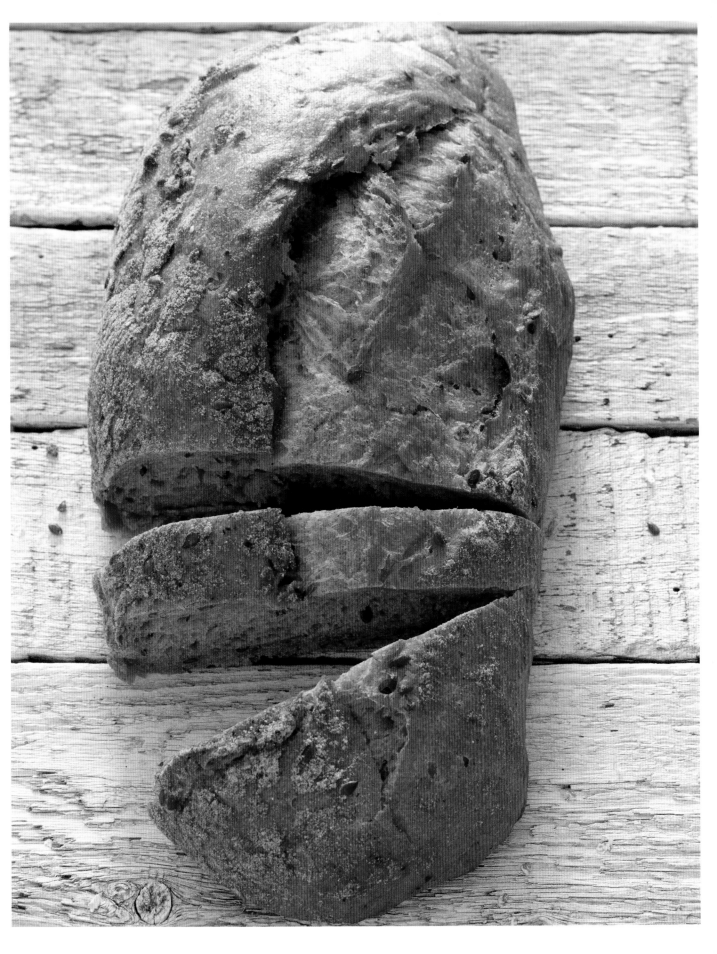

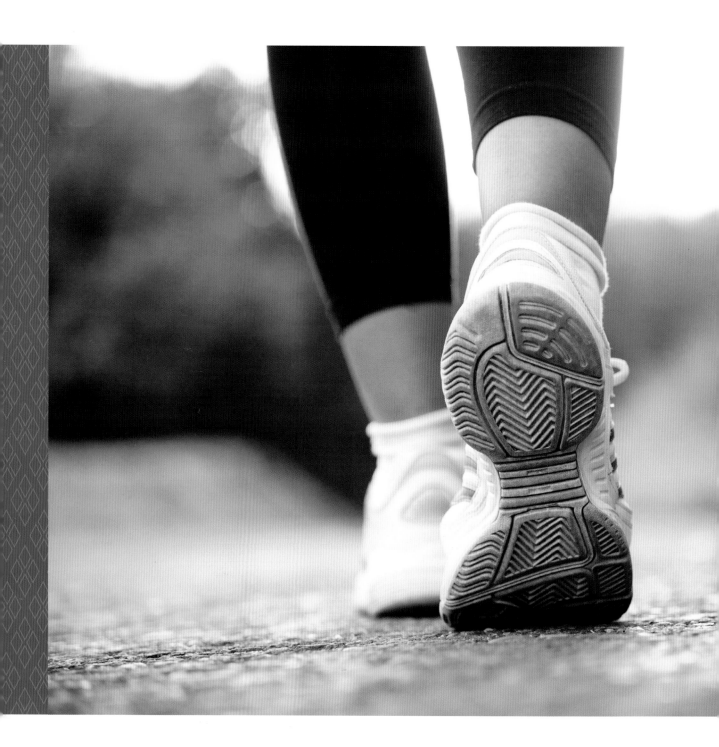

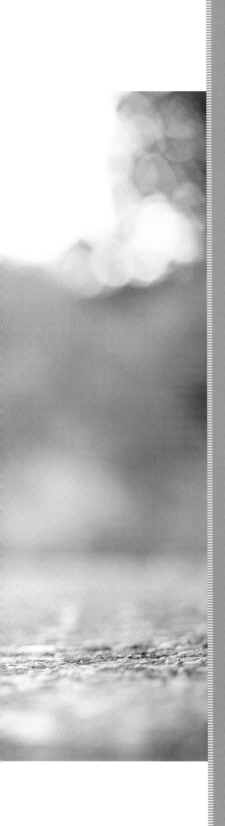

LOSING WEIGHT, KEEPING IT OFF, AND STAYING ACTIVE

Liz's 15 Best Tips for a Healthy Body Weight

WOULD YOU LIKE to achieve and maintain a healthy body weight for the rest of your life? Most of us would. I wish I could tell you that there was some miracle diet or magic pill that could make this happen. Sadly, I don't know of such a thing. What I do know, however, is that if you follow these 15 tips, your chance of success will increase significantly. The advice may seem simple, but it's based on science. Sometimes the simplest ideas still make the most sense.

1. Don't gain it in the first place!

I call this the million-dollar secret to maintaining a healthy body weight. It's by far the most important rule to follow. The key is to pay attention. Notice when your pants start to get tight or the number on the scale starts to inch higher. Once you notice, do something about it right away. Adjust your eating and add more activity to your day. Do whatever it takes to stop the weight-gain train. Why? Preventing weight gain is 100% easier than losing the weight once it's arrived.

2. Don't follow a diet you hate.

Don't follow some crazy, restrictive meal plan that sets you up for failure. If you do, chances are you'll only follow it for about as long as you can stand it, which won't be long. It also sets you up for an unhealthy relationship with food. The best eating plans are designed around healthy foods, but healthy foods that you enjoy! The more customized your plan is to your likes, dislikes, and lifestyle, the more likely it will become a regular part of your life. Achieving a healthy body weight for life requires an eating plan you can follow for life, too.

3. Follow the one-hour rule.

People often resist this rule: Get one hour of exercise a day. That's correct, *one full hour every single day.* If you are doing less than that you will find it challenging to keep your waistline in check, especially as you age. You don't have to do the whole hour at one time, but you do have to commit to getting a full 60 minutes total before the day is through. Do something that gets your heart beating, such as a fast-paced walk. Lift weights at least two to three times a week if you can. The more muscle you have, the more calories you burn, even at rest. Choose activities that you enjoy and that fit into your lifestyle—you'll be more likely to stick with them. Few factors are as strongly associated with obesity as lack of physical activity.

4. Don't say "what the heck."

A consistently healthy body weight requires a consistent eating plan. Take "what the heck" out of your vocabulary. No more "what the heck" it's the weekend or "what the heck" it's the holidays or "what the heck" my cousin Nancy is coming to visit. Too many "what the hecks" and your healthy eating plan goes out the window along with your healthy waistline. I'm not saying don't ever indulge. I'm just saying that the research is clear: Smart people make healthy choices not just some of the time, but most of the time.

5. Learn to manage your emotions.

If you don't know how to manage your emotions in a healthy way, psychologists say that you had better learn and fast. Many people eat because they are bored, stressed, tired, lonely, or unhappy. The result: Emotional eaters have waistlines that expand with their emotions. Don't let that be you! Learn healthy ways to manage your emotions that don't involve food, such as meditation, exercise, or calling a friend. If you need professional help, get it! It's also a good idea to keep a food diary (online or off). Track how often you eat, what you eat, and why you eat. You will be amazed at what you discover. Studies show that people who keep track of eating behaviours are more successful at changing them.

6. Make it easy to eat healthy.

Unfortunately, we live in a toxic food environment where it is easy, if not irresistible, to eat high-fat, high-sugar, calorie-rich foods each and every day. These foods surround us every waking moment and on every street corner. Keep your home and work environment junk-free so healthy eating is the easy thing to do. Our food environment affects our food choices much more than most of us realize.

7. All calories count.

All calories count. Whether you follow a low-fat, low-carb, or high-protein diet doesn't really matter in the long run. What does matter is how many calories you put in your mouth each day. You don't need to be an obsessed calorie counter (life is supposed to be fun!), but you do need to educate yourself about where your calories are coming from and choose accordingly. Simply reducing your portion sizes goes a long way. Eating lots of fruits and vegetables is also key to success.

8. Don't drink your calories.

There is clear and consistent evidence that people do not compensate for the added calories they consume in beverages by reducing their intake of other foods. Eat your calories and drink low-fat milk and no-calorie beverages such as tea and water. Can drinking water actually help you lose weight? Research says yes, especially if

FOOD *for* THOUGHT

"The amount of resources that have gone into studying 'what' to eat is incredible, and years of research indicate that it doesn't really matter, as long as overall calories are reduced. What does matter is 'how' to eat, as well as other things in lifestyle interventions, such as physical activity and supportive behaviours that help people stay on track in the long term."

BRADLEY APPELHANS, PHD, Rush University Medical Center in Chicago

water is replacing calorie-containing beverages like soft drinks. Drinking more water is linked to a significant reduction in body weight, waist circumference, and an improvement in blood pressure. Drinking water instead of other beverages also results in greater fat oxidation because it does not stimulate insulin.

9. Dine at home most of the time.

If you eat in restaurants, especially fast-food restaurants, your waistline will likely pay the price. Dining out and expanding waistlines go hand in hand—study after study has found this to be true. I don't suggest that you never dine out, but if you do, be a wise diner. The more often you eat out, the wiser you need to be.

10. Non-stop snacking is not allowed.

We are a nation of snackers. We snack all day long, to the point that many of us don't know what it feels like to be hungry any more. These snacks are killing us! Be a smart snacker: Plan ahead. Eat small snacks, about 100 to 200 calories or less a few times a day. Eat healthy snacks (fruits and vegetables). Be especially wary of late-night snacks—they're the kind most people simply don't need!

11. Make it a habit.

Habits are now considered one of the most powerful predictors of eating behaviour. Many dietary programs fail because people return to their old habits. Small,

concrete healthy changes give good long-term results. The following five tips have been shown to be highly effective:

1. Keep kitchen counters clear of all foods EXCEPT the healthy ones.

2. Never eat directly from a package—always portion food out into a dish.

3. Avoid going for more than three to four hours without having something small to eat.

4. Put down your utensils between bites to slow down your eating.

5. Eat something for breakfast, at home, within the first hour of waking up.

Commit to each new habit for a full month. It's more likely to become a lifelong routine that way.

12. Get some sleep!

Significant research shows that inadequate sleep makes managing your weight much harder. Adults who get less than six hours of sleep a night are about 55% more likely to be overweight. Lack of sleep can slow metabolism and change hormone levels so that you feel hungrier and eat more (about 300 calories more!). Total sleep time and quality of sleep can even predict how much fat people lose in a weight-loss program.

13. Don't eat these four foods.

When Harvard University researchers looked at the eating habits of over 120,000 men and women over a period of 20 years, they found that four foods were strongly linked to weight gain: french fries, potato chips, sugar-sweetened beverages (primarily soft drinks), and meat (red meat and processed meat). Which foods were linked to healthier waistlines? More natural, whole foods: fruits, vegetables, nuts, whole grains, and yogurt. Make food choices that are good for your health and good for your waistline, too!

14. Don't set lofty goals.

When people set lofty weight-loss goals (10, 20, or 30-plus pounds/4.5, 9, or 13.5-plus kg) and then don't make progress quickly, they believe it's not achievable. Breaking goals down into smaller, more manageable, short-term targets (losing 1 or 2 pounds/500 g to 1 kg a week) can lead to a better chance of success. It's also important to celebrate your mini-successes (not with food!) before getting ready for the next mini-goal.

15. Focus on what you get, get support, and don't give up.

It's important to focus on what you get by eating healthy, not on what you give up. Never say "I have to eat this" or "I can't eat that." Instead say "I choose to eat this" or "I choose not to eat that."

Don't be afraid to get help. See a dietitian or join a program with a proven track record of success, such as Weight Watchers. In a recent study people lost twice as much weight with Weight Watchers than with standard care, such as a family doctor. An independent panel of 22 experts also gave Weight Watchers the gold award for "Best Weight-Loss Diet" (Jenny Craig came in second).

Don't give up! Achieving a healthy body weight can be challenging, especially in the world we live in. Persist in your efforts. The benefits are many. You'll feel better, look better, be able to do more, and slash your risk of heart disease, diabetes, cancer, osteoarthritis, and more!

P.S. Good luck on your journey! I know you can do this!

FOOD *for* THOUGHT

"The proximal cause of obesity is bad use of feet and forks—too many calories and not enough exercise, an energy balance issue. The root cause for most of us is everything about modern living—the availability of tasty, glow-in-the-dark foods, the marketing of food, every device so you don't use your muscles. Sometimes, it's psychological—trauma in childhood, major self-esteem issues, and depression—when food is a Band-Aid. Unless you treat those problems, the dependency on food doesn't go away."

DAVID L. KATZ, MD,
Director of the Yale
Griffin Prevention
Research Center

LESSON LEARNED

To maintain a healthy body weight you should avoid fad diets, drinking your calories, and eating for emotional reasons. Commit to one hour of physical activity daily, be consistent with healthy habits, and keep your home and work environment free of unhealthy foods. Limit dining out, stop endless snacking, and get enough sleep. Most importantly, do your best not to gain excess weight in the first place. Prevention really is the name of the game!

Lack of Exercise Can Kill You

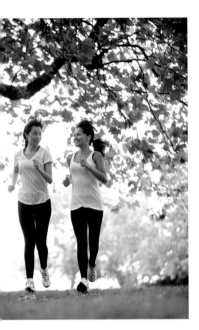

PHYSICAL ACTIVITY SHOULD be a priority in your life every single day. No ifs, no buts, no maybes. The benefits are simply too life changing and miraculous. To ignore this advice is to neglect and abandon your health in the worst way. In fact, some doctors believe that lack of exercise is so harmful to health that it should be treated as a medical condition, just like heart disease or diabetes. This makes sense. Lack of physical activity is strongly linked to pretty much every major health problem there is. If you want to be healthy, you have to be active. You have to spend less time in your car, less time at your computer, and less time in front of the television. The human body was designed to move! Every single cell (and I mean every single one, no exceptions) is happier, healthier, and more joyful when your body is in motion on a regular basis.

ONE MILLION BENEFITS AND COUNTING

The National Institute of Aging has said "if exercise were a drug, it would be the most prescribed medicine in the world." That's because the list of benefits that come with it are truly never-ending. At any age, regular physical activity significantly improves your enjoyment and satisfaction with life. Two of the most vital organs in your body—your heart and brain—absolutely love exercise. It reduces your risk of having a heart attack or stroke and protects you from injury should either one occur. Physical activity is central to the prevention and management of type 2 diabetes. It enhances sensitivity to insulin (less insulin is required to move sugar out of the blood and into the cells) and lessens the many complications associated with this disease, including an increased risk of death. It also helps prevent cancer and is good for bones, blood pressure, and a strong immune system. When regularly active you sleep better, look better, and definitely feel better. It buffers you from stress. Without it, losing weight—and especially keeping the weight off—is next to impossible, as is reducing your risk of dangerous belly or abdominal fat. If you want the ultimate anti-aging tool, keeping your body in motion also slows down and prevents deterioration that would otherwise occur.

POST-MEAL WALKING IS GOOD FOR YOU

In research from Washington University School of Public Health, older adults at risk for diabetes who took a 15-minute walk after each meal improved their blood sugar levels. Three short walks after eating worked better to control blood sugar levels than one 45-minute walk in the morning or evening. Walking helps clear sugar from the blood stream, especially when done within about 30 minutes of the last meal (a time when sugar starts to flood the bloodstream).

WALK AWAY THE BLUES

The World Health Organization estimates that depression will be the second leading cause of incapacitating disease by 2020. Reducing our risk is important. Researchers from the University of Gothenburg in Sweden reviewed 15 studies to determine the effect of exercise on depression. They found that exercise had a "significant, large overall effect" and that it was particularly successful in people with mild to moderate depression who were motivated enough to get moving.

Physical activity reduces depression risk in a multitude of ways, including releasing "feel-good" chemicals in the brain (neurotransmitters and endorphins). It can cut the risk of depression by as much as 50% and is a viable alternative to anti-depressant drugs. All types of activity have been found to be effective, including aerobic activity, yoga, and resistance training. It also shows great promise in those who are at greatest risk for depression, such as the elderly.

THE CANCER–ACTIVITY CONNECTION

The American Institute of Cancer Research says that if you want to significantly reduce your risk of cancer, be active every day in any way for at least 30 minutes. Regular activity is linked to a much lower risk of many types of cancer, including breast, colon, prostate, and endometrium. Staying active helps you maintain a healthy body weight (excess weight is one of the most significant risk factors for cancer). It also protects you by keeping hormone levels healthy, your immune system strong, and inflammation at bay. Those who are active during childhood are also less likely to develop cancer down the road.

MOVE MORE, SLEEP MORE, SLEEP BETTER!

Good-quality sleep has an incredible impact on your overall health and well-being. It affects how you feel each day and significantly decreases your risk of many diseases, including obesity. Regular physical activity helps you fall asleep faster, sleep more deeply, and stay asleep longer. It's an effective and healthy alternative to sleeping pills.

PHYSICAL ACTIVITY AND THE COMMON COLD

One of the most significant factors influencing how often you get sick (like

FOOD *for* THOUGHT
"Leave all the afternoon for exercise and recreation, which are as necessary as reading. I will rather say more necessary because health is worth more than learning."
THOMAS JEFFERSON, Third President of the United States

catching a cold or flu) and the severity of your symptoms is whether you are physically active on a regular basis. Regular, moderate activity significantly strengthens your immune system and cuts your risk of illness by as much as 50%. It boosts the activity of immune cells, including "natural killer" cells, which are potent weapons against viruses that lead to infection.

AGING AND BRAIN HEALTH

Regular physical activity has an incredible impact on the aging process. There is no substitute for it. It helps preserve lean muscle, reduces the risk of falling or injury, and is critical to a strong and healthy heart. It is especially important to the health of the aging brain. The research supporting this is strong, consistent, and robust. Regular activity helps preserve memory, along with the ability to pay attention and make decisions. It promotes the growth of new brain cells and enhances both brain cell communication and survival. Your risk of dementia, including Alzheimer's disease, as well as developing small brain lesions (sometimes referred to as "silent strokes") are also significantly reduced.

STOP YOUR BRAIN FROM SHRINKING

Researchers from the Centre for Cognitive Aging in Edinburgh report that regular exercise, such as walking several times a week, in old age is even better for brain health than engaging in mental

or social activities. This study involved over 600 men and women over the age of 70 over a three-year period. MRI brain scans found that regular physical activity helped to prevent brain shrinkage, which means there was less brain cell death. It also helped preserve the intricate wiring that transmits messages in the brain.

THE ANTI-AGING IMPACT

At the ends of our DNA (the blueprint our cells use to reproduce) there are protective caps called "telomeres." Longer telomeres are linked to younger cells and a longer life. Exercise promotes healthy aging by protecting and preventing shortening of telomeres. It's like changing your biological clock. You still age, but not as quickly. Have your running shoes on yet?

LESS HOUSEWORK, BIGGER WAISTLINES!

About 50 years ago women spent a lot more time doing housework—cleaning, cooking, and doing laundry. These are all activities that burn calories. Today women spend far more time sitting. The result? Researchers from the University of South Carolina compared activity levels of women in 1965 with those in 2010. They found that women today burn as much as 360 fewer calories a day than women in the past. No wonder our waistlines are expanding. This doesn't mean you have to clean your house more, but you do have to make the effort to be more active each and every day.

HOW ACTIVE DO YOU NEED TO BE?

The Canadian Society for Exercise Physiology recommends that adults accumulate at least 150 minutes (2.5 hours) per week of moderate- to vigorous-intensity aerobic physical activity in bouts of 10 minutes or more. They also recommend muscle- and bone-strengthening activities using major muscle groups (lifting weights or doing push-ups or sit-ups) at least twice a week. Children and teens are encouraged to get at least one hour of activity a day. The Canadian guidelines are consistent with other major health organizations around the world, including the World Health Organization and the US Department of Health and Human Services Guidelines for Americans. The majority of both adults and children today do not meet these guidelines. For optimal weight control (loss or maintenance) being active for at least 60 minutes a day should be your goal.

RUNNING NOT REQUIRED

Joan Rivers said, "The first time I see a jogger smiling, I'll consider it." I myself have always preferred walking to running, although I definitely walk at a very brisk pace. The good news is both walking and running appear to provide similar health benefits. Researchers from Lawrence Berkeley National Laboratory in California compared the health of 33,000 runners to almost 16,000 walkers over a period of almost six years. They found that walking briskly lowered the risk of high blood pressure, high cholesterol, and diabetes as much as running, as long as the amount of energy expended (calories burned) was the same (walkers, therefore, had to walk longer to burn the same amount of calories). They also found that the more each ran and walked, the greater the health benefits for both. This is great news! Walking is the most accessible, prevalent, and well-liked physical activity. Just make sure that you walk at a fairly brisk pace. Other research has shown that walking pace is more important to health than walking distance.

REGULAR WALKERS REMAIN INDEPENDENT

Research from the University of Georgia reports that older adults who walk regularly (about three times a week for about 40 minutes at a time) cut their risk of disability and increase their likelihood of maintaining independence by over 40%.

10,000 STEPS PER DAY

If you want to be more active, get a pedometer. A pedometer is a handy little gadget that clips onto your clothing and measures how many steps you take each day. Researchers from Stanford University in California reviewed 26 studies and found that pedometers encourage people to take at least 2,000 extra steps a day. That's significant! The use of pedometers was also linked to significant decreases in body weight and blood pressure. Having a step goal (10,000 steps daily is the

> FOOD *for* THOUGHT
> "Extra fat that accumulates around the abdomen goes by many names: beer belly, spare tire, love handles, apple shape, middle-age spread, and the more technical 'abdominal obesity.' No matter what the name, it is the shape of risk. Abdominal obesity increases the risk of heart attack, stroke, diabetes, erectile dysfunction, and other woes."
> **HARVEY B. SIMON, MD, Editor, Harvard Health Publications**

recommended standard) was also found to be important. If you don't already have a pedometer, go get one!

INTERVAL TRAINING IS GOOD FOR YOU

Short on time? Although high-intensity interval training is not for everyone (some people just don't like it), research shows it provides significant health benefits. Interval training is an exercise strategy that alternates short, intense periods of cardio (like sprinting as fast as you can for one or two minutes) with less-intense recovery periods (like walking at a more moderate pace for five minutes). It appears to be particularly beneficial for heart health, fat burning, and blood sugar control. Just 20 to 30 minutes of this type of activity is good for health. Perhaps you should give it a try?

I LOVE PLAYING HOCKEY!

I shouldn't have to say this because it's so obvious, but I will: When it comes to physical activity, finding an activity you enjoy and one that fits into your lifestyle is critical. When I was a new mother I joined a gym that had a daycare. When my kids got bigger and my work schedule became more demanding having a treadmill and weights in my basement was ideal. Today I hike almost daily in the ravine near my home and office. It's convenient, I love being in nature, and I love hiking. Playing hockey in the winter and kayaking in the summer are both activities I enjoy. Dancing any time (including in my living room every single day!) is another way I stay active. Find what works for you and then do it!

EVERYTHING COUNTS!

Take the stairs instead of the escalator. Rake the leaves instead of using a leaf blower. Walk into the store instead of going through the drive-thru. Every single time you move your body, your body says thank you. Make movement a regular part of your life.

LESSON LEARNED

Regular physical activity is essential for optimal health and enjoyment of life. Lack of activity creates disease and shortens lives—big time! Make every day an active day. The human body was designed to move.

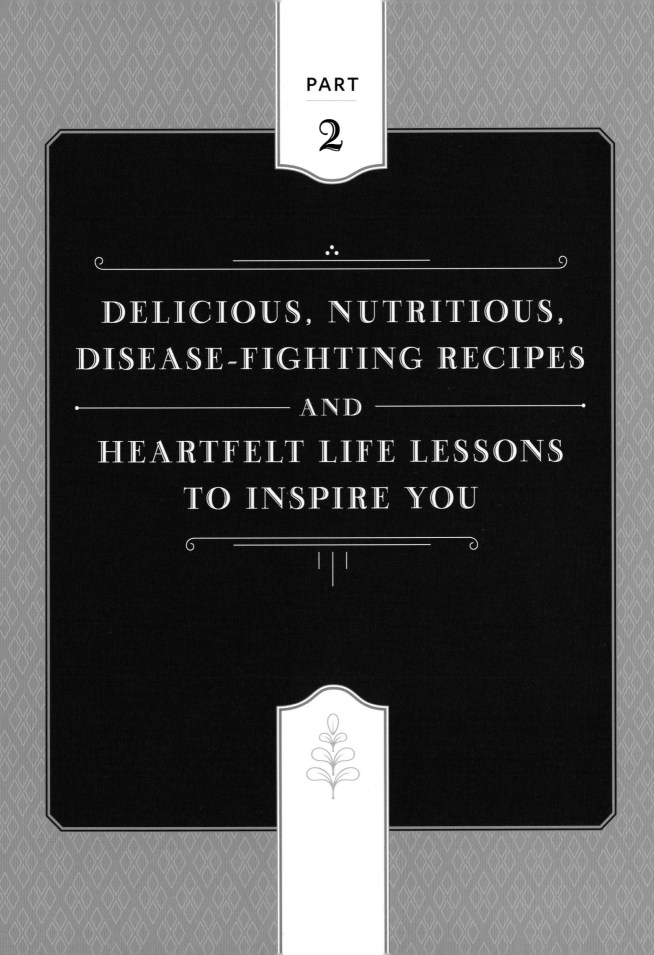

PART

2

DELICIOUS, NUTRITIOUS,
DISEASE-FIGHTING RECIPES
— AND —
HEARTFELT LIFE LESSONS
TO INSPIRE YOU

WELCOME TO THE recipe and life lesson section of the book! The recipes are totally delicious and loaded with powerful, health-protective ingredients, including berries, dark leafy greens, whole grains, beans, and omega-3-rich fish. There are soups, salads, side dishes, main-course meals, healthy snacks, and great smoothie recipes, too. I even left room for chocolate, including a decadent chocolate cake (page 289) you definitely don't want to miss! Best of all, every single recipe comes with a heartfelt life lesson. These lessons mirror my own evolution and, in many ways, my greatest passion: to live my life better and more wisely and to approach each day with a little more love, gratitude, and kindness than the day before. My goal is to inspire you to do the same. Being healthy is not enough. I want you to be happy, too! I encourage you to read each lesson every time you make a recipe. Cooking time, after all, is a great time for reflection. Here's to delicious, healthy eating *and* living your best life!

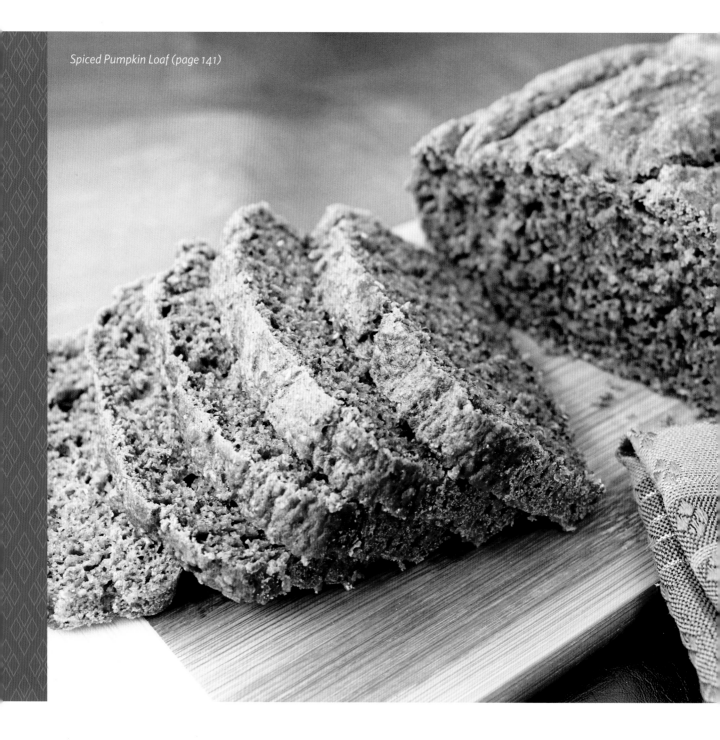

Spiced Pumpkin Loaf (page 141)

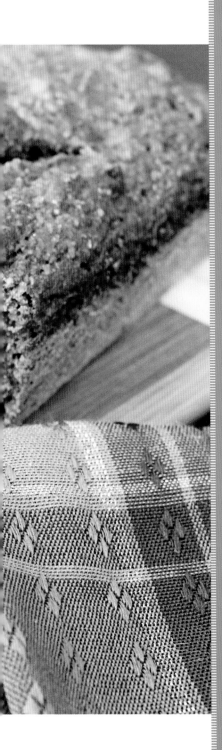

MUFFINS, LOAVES, PANCAKES, AND WAFFLES

*A life lesson comes with
every recipe. Enjoy!*

ANIMALS TEACH US HOW TO LIVE

> "Animals are reliable, many full of love, true in their affections, predictable in their actions, grateful, and loyal. Difficult standards for people to live up to." **ALFRED A. MONTAPERT**

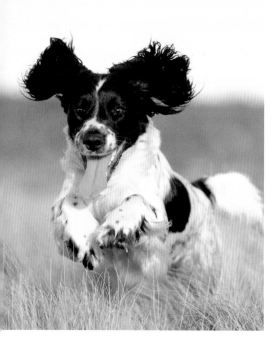

I F YOU COULD be any animal, which would you choose? I can't pick just one—it's too limiting. I've decided I'd like to be a duck, a tortoise, a chimpanzee, a lion, an owl, an eagle, and a dog. A little much, I know, but that's just me.

As a duck, I'd let all the stuff that really doesn't matter—which is most stuff —just roll off my back. As a tortoise, I'd slow down. It's only when I slow down that I'm able to see the beauty that surrounds me. As a chimpanzee, I'd embrace fun and swing through the treetops of life whenever I got the chance. As a lion, I'd have so much courage I'd do even the things that scare me the most. As an owl, I'd grow to be wise simply by observing my surroundings. As an eagle, I'd soar to new heights and achieve things I never imagined possible. As a dog—and perhaps this is the most important one—I'd love the people who matter most in my life just as they are and I'd be the best friend they ever had.

LESSON LEARNED

Animals teach us to slow down, live in the moment, have fun, be brave, be wise, reach higher, and love deeply without limits. Do your best to be more animal-like today.

Apple Pie Muffins

If you love apple pie, then you'll love these muffins. Made with 100% whole-wheat flour, they are chock full of healthy ingredients, including apples, cinnamon, and nutmeg. Don't peel the apples before you dice them: the skin is loaded with antioxidants. Granny Smith apples, in particular, are antioxidant all-stars. These muffins taste best right out of the oven. Enjoy! **MAKES 12 MUFFINS**

1. Preheat the oven to 375°F (190°C).
2. In a medium bowl, combine all the dry ingredients.
3. In a small bowl, whisk together all the wet ingredients.
4. Add the wet ingredients to the dry ingredients and mix until just combined.
5. Divide the batter evenly into 12 paper-lined or well-greased muffin cups. Bake for 20 to 25 minutes or until the tops are firm to the touch.

PER MUFFIN 169 calories • 5.5 g fat • 0.7 g saturated fat •
28 g carbohydrates • 13 g sugars • 3.5 g fibre • 3 g protein • 116 mg sodium

DRY INGREDIENTS

2 cups (500 mL) whole-wheat flour

2 Granny Smith apples, finely diced (leave skin on)

1 Tbsp (15 mL) ground cinnamon

1 Tbsp (15 mL) ground nutmeg

2 tsp (10 mL) baking powder

½ tsp (2.5 mL) baking soda

WET INGREDIENTS

½ cup (125 mL) low-fat milk (skim or 1%)

½ cup (125 mL) orange juice

½ cup (125 mL) pure maple syrup

¼ cup (60 mL) canola oil

1 tsp (5 mL) pure vanilla extract

1 tsp (5 mL) freshly grated lemon peel (zest)

1 omega-3 egg

THE JOY OF REALIZING A DREAM

> "Go confidently in the direction of your dreams. Live the life you have imagined." **HENRY DAVID THOREAU**

IMAGINE CROSSING AFRICA from north to south and covering almost 7,500 miles (about 12,000 km) on your bike (and I don't mean a motor bike!) over a period of four months. The trip is called Tour d'Afrique, and it is considered a test of the mind, body, and bike. Bev Coburn, the sister of a woman I play hockey with, completed this challenge in 2012 at the age of 62. From sunrise to sunset, she rode through every condition imaginable, often in very remote areas. Bev had dreamed of doing this trip for many years. She thought it would be the trip of a lifetime—and it truly was! She loved the physical exertion. She loved the unique personality and breathtaking beauty of each of the 10 countries she travelled through. She loved doing something that was so challenging. It was frightening at times, but always amazing. She learned how to adapt to every type of person and situation imaginable. She discovered that how she thinks and does things is not always the way other people think and do things. The best part, she explained, was experiencing "pure joy." When did she feel this joy the most? Although she did this trip with a group of 42 other people, much of each day was spent riding on her own, all by herself. Just her and her bike and the vast, glorious land all around her. Talk about joy! At times she wanted to pinch herself. "Is this really me? Am I really doing this?" Yes, it was her and she was doing it! How about you? What's your dream and are you doing it?

LESSON LEARNED

Dreams are meant to be followed. Have the courage to follow yours. Do things that challenge you, scare you, and make you feel alive. You've got one life to live: Make it a great one!

Wild Blueberry Muffins

Berries are disease-fighting superstars. Making them a regular part of your eating plan is one of the wisest decisions you can make. These 100% whole-grain muffins are loaded with antioxidant-rich wild blueberries. They're incredibly moist and tasty, and the combination of lemon, blueberries, and maple is really wonderful. Enjoy! **MAKES 12 MUFFINS**

1. Preheat the oven to 375°F (190°C).
2. In a medium bowl, combine the oats, milk, and lemon zest and juice. Let sit.
3. In a small bowl, combine the flour, cinnamon, baking powder, and baking soda.
4. In another small bowl, whisk together the maple syrup, oil, and egg.
5. Transfer the ingredients from the two small bowls to the medium bowl. Stir until just combined. Carefully fold in the blueberries.
6. Divide the batter evenly into 12 paper-lined or well-greased muffin cups. Bake for 20 to 25 minutes or until the tops are firm to the touch.

PER MUFFIN 151 calories · 6 g fat · 0.6 g saturated fat ·
23 g carbohydrates · 2.5 g fibre · 3 g protein · 116 mg sodium

1 cup (250 mL) large-flake oats

¾ cup (185 mL) low-fat milk (skim or 1%)

Grated peel (zest) and juice of 1 lemon

1 cup (250 mL) whole-wheat flour

1 Tbsp (15 mL) ground cinnamon

2 tsp (10 mL) baking powder

½ tsp (2.5 mL) baking soda

½ cup (125 mL) pure maple syrup

¼ cup (60 mL) canola oil

1 omega-3 egg

1½ cups (375 mL) wild blueberries (fresh or frozen)

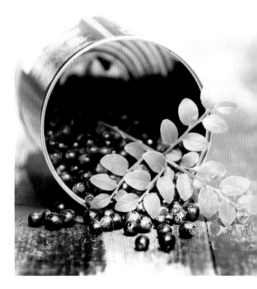

TONY ROBBINS INSPIRED ME... WHO INSPIRES YOU?

> "Our chief want is someone who will inspire us to be what we know we could be." **RALPH WALDO EMERSON**

THIS IS THE fourth book that I have written. My first book, *When in Doubt, Eat Broccoli! (But Leave Some Room for Chocolate)*, came out in 1998. People often ask me what inspired me to write a book in the first place. My answer is Tony Robbins, the motivational speaker and life coach. I used to listen to his tapes and read his books. He, along with other self-help gurus, inspired me to think bigger, follow my dreams, and take action. In fact, a few years after my first book was published, I had the wonderful opportunity of seeing Tony Robbins speak live in Toronto. When he first came running out onto the stage, I started to cry. I never anticipated such a reaction. In that moment I realized just how grateful I was to him and all that he had brought to my life. He inspired me to take steps I might not have otherwise taken. How about you? Who moves you? Do your friends encourage you to follow your dreams? Do the books you read urge you think bigger and bolder? Do the television shows or movies you watch push you to reach higher? It's been said that we become who we spend time with. How are you spending your time? Get inspired by spending time with those people who lift you up and make you want to do more, achieve more, and be more.

LESSON LEARNED

To live an inspired life, fill your life with people and situations that inspire you. It is often through others that we get the courage, strength, wisdom, and drive to dream bigger, reach higher, and truly stand in our power and who we are meant to be.

High-Fibre Muffins with Raspberries and Flax

We could all use more fibre in our diets. It's great for gut health, lowers blood cholesterol, and helps keep your appetite in check. Here's a totally delicious way to get more of it into your eating plan. These yummy muffins are made with whole-wheat flour and loaded with high-fibre ingredients: flaxseeds, sunflower seeds, raspberries, and dates. You get 7 grams of fibre per muffin along with a whole lot of great nutrition.

P.S. I recently received a lovely note from a friend who tried these muffins. She said they lasted a day and everyone—her kids, in-laws, and husband—loved them. Enjoy! **MAKES 12 MUFFINS**

1. Preheat the oven to 375°F (190°C).
2. In a medium bowl, combine the flour, flaxseeds, sunflower seeds, cinnamon, cloves, baking powder, and baking soda. Set aside.
3. In a blender, blend the orange juice, milk, dates, egg, and maple syrup until smooth. (You can also mix the ingredients in a small bowl using a hand-held blender. Pre-chop the dates if using this option.)
4. Add the wet ingredients to the dry ingredients and stir until combined. Fold in the raspberries.
5. Divide the batter evenly into 12 paper-lined or well-greased muffin cups. Bake for 20 to 25 minutes or until the tops are firm to the touch.

TIP
- You can buy flaxseeds pre-ground or grind them yourself in a clean coffee grinder.

PER MUFFIN 188 calories • 6 g fat • 1 g saturated fat • 30 g carbohydrates • 14 g sugars • 7 g fibre • 6 g protein • 118 mg sodium

1 cup (250 mL) whole-wheat flour

1 cup (250 mL) ground flaxseeds

½ cup (125 mL) unsalted sunflower seeds (raw or roasted)

1 Tbsp (15 mL) ground cinnamon

1 tsp (5 mL) ground cloves

2 tsp (10 mL) baking powder

½ tsp (2.5 mL) baking soda

1 cup (250 mL) orange juice

½ cup (125 mL) low-fat milk (skim or 1%)

1 cup (250 mL) dates

1 omega-3 egg

¼ cup (60 mL) pure maple syrup

1½ cups (375 mL) raspberries (fresh or frozen)

NATURE HEALS LIKE NO OTHER

"Keep close to Nature's heart . . . and break clear away, once in a while, and climb a mountain or spend a week in the woods. Wash your spirit clean." **JOHN MUIR**

WHEN MY DAUGHTER Chelsea was about five years old we went to visit my brother who lives on a farm. While we were there I asked her whether she would rather live in the city or the country. "The country," she replied. When I asked her why, she responded, "It just feels good!" These are wise words. After returning home from hiking the West Coast Trail, I came to the conclusion that human beings were not created to live our lives inside four walls and a ceiling. The concrete jungle is not our true home. Outside and in nature is where we find true peace, true calm, and real beauty. It's where we connect deeply to ourselves, to a power beyond ourselves, and to what matters. It's where we heal. Although I still live much of my life indoors, I make it a priority to spend time outdoors every single day. When I'm not travelling, I hike in the ravine near my house. It has a winding river, many tall and majestic trees, and some incredible lookouts. There is not one single day spent in that ravine that I don't feel incredible gratitude for all that it brings to my life. How often do you spend time in nature? Do you let it touch you, calm you, and heal your soul?

LESSON LEARNED

Nature is among the greatest of all gifts. Appreciate it, take care of it, and spend time with this gift. It will enrich you and touch your soul as few other things can.

Awesome Maple Banana Bread

Try my homemade maple banana bread. It's nutritious and awesomely delicious! Be sure to use 100% pure maple syrup—it's a significant source of antioxidants and nothing beats the taste of the real thing. Flaxseeds are an excellent source of omega-3 fats, fibre, and cancer-fighting plant compounds called lignans. Enjoy! **MAKES 1 LOAF**

1. Preheat the oven to 350°F (175°C).
2. In a medium bowl, combine all of the dry ingredients.
3. In a small bowl, combine all of the wet ingredients.
4. Add the wet ingredients to the dry ingredients and mix until just combined.
5. Pour the mixture into a lightly greased 9- × 5-inch (2 L) loaf pan. Bake for 45 to 55 minutes or until a toothpick inserted into the centre of the loaf comes out clean. Let cool in the pan for about 5 minutes, then turn out onto a wire rack to cool completely.

TIP
- You can buy flaxseeds pre-ground or grind them yourself in a clean coffee grinder.

PER SLICE (ABOUT ½ INCH/1 CM THICK) 139 calories • 4.5 g fat • 0.5 g saturated fat • 23 g carbohydrates • 11 g sugars • 2.5 g fibre • 2.5 g protein • 93 mg sodium

DRY INGREDIENTS

1½ cups (375 mL) whole-wheat flour

½ cup (125 mL) ground flaxseeds

2 tsp (10 mL) ground cinnamon

1 tsp (5 mL) baking powder

1 tsp (5 mL) baking soda

WET INGREDIENTS

4 very ripe medium bananas, mashed

¾ cup (185 mL) pure maple syrup

¼ cup (60 mL) canola oil

1 tsp (5 mL) pure vanilla extract

1 omega-3 egg, beaten

DARE TO LOOK... AT WHAT YOU DON'T WANT TO LOOK AT

> "You will find peace not by trying to escape your problems, but by confronting them courageously. You will find peace not in denial, but in victory." **J. DONALD WALTERS**

MY MARRIAGE WAS falling apart long before I was willing to look at the fact that my marriage was falling apart. I didn't want to look. I had decided that my children would never experience that nasty thing called divorce. I had decided that my kids would get the fairy-tale ending, the kind that all kids want: a mom and a dad who love each other and stay together until the end. I wanted this story so much that I refused to look at my reality. By the time I finally looked, many years had passed. My marriage wasn't just over, it was done and I was really unhappy. You pay a huge price for the things you don't look at. The longer you don't look, the bigger the price. It takes tremendous courage, strength, and honesty to look. The things that are the hardest and most painful to look at are usually the things that need our attention most. We often don't like what we see. Looking, however, is the only way to grow. It's the only way to make your life all that you want it to be. Are there any parts of your life—marriage, kids, work, self—that you need to look at? Dare to look. Dare to live.

LESSON LEARNED
Don't deny your reality. It's only by looking honestly at your life that you can make it all you want it to be.

Spiced Pumpkin Loaf

When my friends invite me for a visit, I ask them, "What would you like me to bring?" They always respond, "Bring your pumpkin loaf!" I guess they like it. This whole-grain loaf is made with whole-wheat flour and lots of antioxidant-rich, health-protective spices. Pumpkin is an exceptional source of beta-carotene. Flaxseeds are rich in fibre, heart-healthy omega-3 fats, as well as cancer-fighting plant compounds called lignans. Enjoy!

MAKES 2 LOAVES

1. Preheat the oven to 350°F (175°C).
2. In a small bowl, combine the milk and lemon juice and let sit for 5 minutes.
3. Meanwhile, in a medium bowl, combine the flour, flaxseeds, ginger, cinnamon, allspice, cloves, baking powder, and baking soda.
4. To the milk and lemon juice mixture, add the pumpkin purée, maple syrup, canola oil, and eggs. Mix well.
5. Add the wet ingredients to the dry ingredients and mix until just combined.
6. Pour equal amounts of the mixture into two lightly greased 9- × 5-inch (2 L) loaf pans. Bake for 50 to 55 minutes or until a toothpick inserted into the centre of each loaf comes out clean. Let cool in the pan for about 5 minutes, then turn out onto a wire rack to cool completely.

TIPS

- To make only one loaf, divide the ingredients in half (you can also make two loaves and freeze one).
- You can buy flaxseeds pre-ground or grind them yourself in a clean coffee grinder.
- For a special presentation, dust each loaf with icing sugar just before serving it to guests.

¾ cup (185 mL) low-fat milk (skim or 1%)

1 Tbsp (15 mL) freshly squeezed lemon juice

2½ cups (625 mL) whole-wheat flour

1 cup (250 mL) ground flaxseeds

2 Tbsp (30 mL) ground ginger

1 Tbsp (15 mL) ground cinnamon

2 tsp (10 mL) ground allspice

2 tsp (10 mL) ground cloves

2 tsp (10 mL) baking powder

2 tsp (10 mL) baking soda

2 cups (500 mL) pumpkin purée

1¼ cups (310 mL) pure maple syrup

⅓ cup (80 mL) canola oil

2 omega-3 eggs

PER SLICE (ABOUT ½ INCH/1 CM THICK) 106 calories • 3.5 g fat • 0.4 g saturated fat • 17 g carbohydrates • 7.5 g sugars • 2 g fibre • 2.5 g protein • 96 mg sodium

WHAT IS A FAMILY?

> "Love makes a family." **GIGI KAESER**

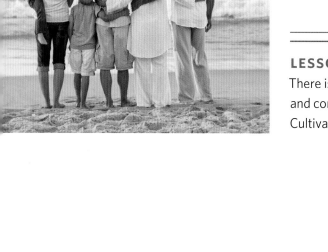

IRECENTLY SPENT A weekend at a cottage with a family I've known most of my life. As I watched them (mom, dad, and three kids who range in age from 17 to 21) interact, I pondered the question "What is a family?" This is my definition: A family is made up of people who are all different yet are bonded together in a very special way. Each person has their own unique interests and personality, yet as a family they stand as one. Sometimes they get along and other times they don't. Sometimes they work together, other times they play together, and then there are times they simply co-exist in the same place, each doing their own thing. However, all families (good families, that is) share three core traits: They love each other, they care about each other, and they respect each other. I was privileged to witness genuine love, caring, and respect all weekend long. It made me truly appreciate the beauty of a family. How beautiful is your family? Is there anything you could be doing to make it even more beautiful?

LESSON LEARNED

There is incredible beauty in a family, including love, caring, respect, and connections that run deep. Honour and appreciate that beauty. Cultivate that beauty in your own family.

Wickedly Wonderful Waffles

Weekends are the perfect time for waffles, especially whole-grain waffles that taste great. If you don't own a waffle iron, perhaps now is a great time to get one. Waffles make breakfast more fun! I love to eat waffles with plenty of fresh berries on top—that way I get berries plus waffle in every bite. The combination is amazing. Enjoy! **SERVES 4**

1. In a medium bowl, combine the dry ingredients.
2. In a small bowl, whisk together the wet ingredients.
3. Add the wet ingredients to the dry ingredients and stir until combined.
4. Preheat the waffle iron. When ready, spray with non-stick vegetable oil. Pour the batter onto the iron. Cook until golden brown. Repeat until the batter is used up.
5. Serve with pure maple syrup and fresh berries (at least ½ cup/125 mL of berries per waffle).

TIP

- You can replace the oats with an equal measure of whole-grain cornmeal. Try both of these delicious options and let me know which one you like best.

PER WAFFLE (WHEN MADE WITH OATS) 237 calories • 12 g fat • 1.5 g saturated fat • 28 g carbohydrate • 5 g fibre • 8 g protein • 191 mg sodium

PER WAFFLE (WHEN MADE WITH CORNMEAL) 251 calories • 11 g fat • 1 g saturated fat • 32 g carbohydrate • 5.5 g fibre • 8 g protein • 195 mg sodium

DRY INGREDIENTS

½ cup (125 mL) whole-wheat flour

½ cup (125 mL) large-flake oats

¼ cup (60 mL) ground flaxseeds

1 Tbsp (15 mL) ground cinnamon

2 tsp (10 mL) baking powder

WET INGREDIENTS

¾ cup (185 mL) low-fat milk (skim or 1%)

2 Tbsp (30 mL) canola oil

1 Tbsp (15 mL) pure maple syrup

½ tsp (2.5 mL) pure vanilla extract

1 omega-3 egg

A GREAT LIFE INCLUDES GREAT MUSIC

"After silence, that which comes nearest to expressing the inexpressible is music." **ALDOUS HUXLEY**

THE OTHER DAY I had lunch with a long-time friend. He told me that his mother had recently lost most of her hearing and that she doesn't like to use hearing aids. As a result, the world for her now is a much quieter place. What does she miss the most? Listening to music. I can understand. Music is a true passion of mine and always has been. When I taught aerobics, I never made any money because I spent it all on the next playlist. When my brother got married, I was the disc jockey at his wedding. For me, planning a party is about planning the music. My daughter recently said that we couldn't have an exchange student live at our house because I play my music too loud (ha ha!). What is it about music that I find so compelling? When it comes right down to it, I think music is an expression of the soul. It makes life and everything in it bigger and brighter. A happy song makes you feel happier. A sad song lets you feel your sadness. A love song allows the love to flow. If you accept the premise that when you *feel* life, you *live* life, then music helps you to live life that much more. Take some time today to listen to and truly appreciate music and how it makes you feel.

LESSON LEARNED

Music makes life bigger, bolder, and definitely more beautiful. It connects you to yourself, to others, and to life itself. Let the music play!

P.S. My website, including my blog, can be found at www.lizpearson.com. Here you'll find my top 10 playlists for all-around great songs, dance songs, slow songs, rock songs, and country songs (www.lizpearson.com/living-a-great-life-includes-listening-to-great-music). Enjoy!

Wild Blueberry Pancakes

I love these whole-grain blueberry pancakes. I made them for the kids on my street and got two thumbs up from each and every taster. My daughter's only comment was that she'd prefer them with chocolate chips instead of blueberries (we have more than one chocolate lover in the family). If you do decide to substitute chocolate chips for berries, only add about ¼ to ½ cup (60 to 125 mL). I do, however, encourage you to try them with berries as well—they are berry delicious! Enjoy! **SERVES 4 TO 5 (MAKES ABOUT 10 SMALL PANCAKES)**

1. In a large bowl, mix together all of the dry ingredients.
2. In a medium bowl, whisk together all of the wet ingredients.
3. Add the wet ingredients to the dry ingredients and stir until just combined. Fold in the blueberries. Set aside for 5 minutes to allow time for the oats to soften.
4. Heat a large non-stick skillet or griddle over medium heat. Spray with non-stick vegetable oil. Pour about ⅓ cup (80 mL) of batter for each pancake. Cook until the bubbles break on top and the bottoms are golden, about 2 minutes. Flip and cook until golden on bottom, about 1 to 2 minutes.
5. Keep warm in the oven or serve immediately with pure maple syrup.

TIP

- You can substitute raspberries or blackberries for the blueberries or use mixed berries, too!

PER PANCAKE (4 INCHES/10 CM IN DIAMETER) 163 calories ▪ 4 g fat ▪ 0.5 g saturated fat ▪ 26 g carbohydrates ▪ 4.5 g sugars ▪ 4 g fibre ▪ 6 g protein ▪ 152 mg sodium

DRY INGREDIENTS

1½ cups (375 mL) whole-wheat flour

1 cup (250 mL) large-flake oats

2 tsp (10 mL) baking powder

2 tsp (10 mL) ground cinnamon

½ tsp (2.5 mL) ground nutmeg

½ tsp (2.5 mL) baking soda

WET INGREDIENTS

1½ cups (375 mL) low-fat milk (skim or 1%)

½ cup (125 mL) orange juice

2 Tbsp (30 mL) canola oil

1 tsp (5 mL) pure vanilla extract

1 omega-3 egg, beaten

1 cup (250 mL) wild blueberries (fresh or frozen)

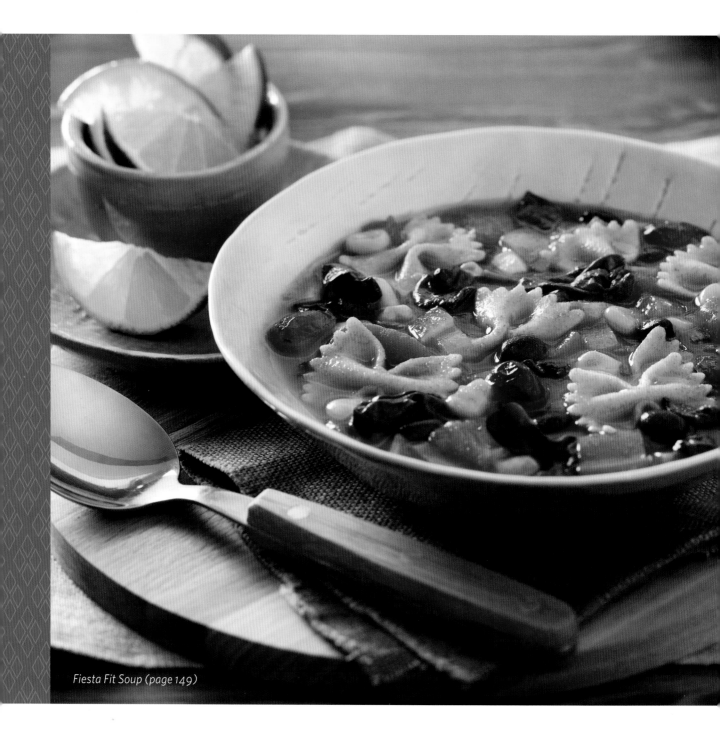

Fiesta Fit Soup (page 149)

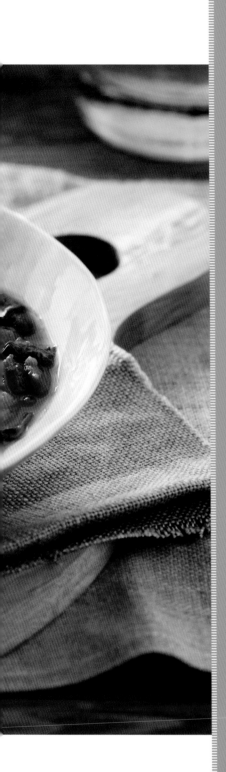

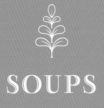

SOUPS

*A life lesson comes with
every recipe. Enjoy!*

THE JOY OF FREEDOM

> "Is freedom anything else than the right to live as we wish? Nothing else." **EPICTETUS**

MICHAEL FISHBACH IS co-founder of the Great Whale Conservancy. Each year he spends two months on the Sea of Cortez photographing and tracking humpback whales. On Valentine's Day 2011, he came across a young whale in the water that was almost dead. It had become completely entangled in a nylon fishing net. Michael and his friends worked steadily to cut the net, piece by piece, away from the whale's body. A few hours later the whale was, once again, free. This is when the show began. Michael and his friends watched as the whale leapt high out of the water and into the air over and over again, performing at least 40 breaches, along with multiple tail lobs, tail slaps, and fin flaps. It was a magnificent show. It appeared to be a show of pure joy and real gratitude—a celebration of what it means to be truly free. It made me think about how much I value my own freedom. Are you free? Do you listen to and follow your own heart? Is your life what you want it to be? Are you doing the things you want to be doing? Are you spending time with those you want to spend time with? Does your life express who you really are and what you're truly capable of? What net entangles and holds you back? Can you cut it away, piece by piece, bit by bit? Will you do the work required? How free do you want to be?

LESSON LEARNED

Freedom is your birthright. It's what you deserve. Work hard to achieve it, sustain it, feel it, and live it. With freedom comes happiness and, more importantly, pure joy.

Fiesta Fit Soup

Imagine a soup that is fast, easy, gives new meaning to the word "delicious," and contains ingredients—whole grains, beans, healthy fats, peppers, and flavonoid-rich fruits and vegetables—that are linked to a lower risk of belly fat. Does it get any better? I don't think so. I helped develop this soup as part of a campaign I worked on with Catelli Healthy Harvest® Whole-grain Pasta. It gets rave reviews and leftovers are great for lunch at the office the next day. I hope you love it as much as I do. Enjoy! SERVES **8**

1. In a large pot over medium heat, heat the oil. Add the onion and red pepper. Sauté for 2 to 3 minutes or until softened.
2. Add the cranberries, garlic, chili powder, cumin, salt, and pepper. Cook, stirring, for 1 minute. Stir in 6 cups (1.5 L) of the broth and the tomatoes; bring to a boil.
3. Stir in the beans, pasta, and corn. Return to a boil and simmer gently, partially covered and stirring occasionally, for 12 minutes or until the pasta is tender.
4. Stir in the remaining 2 cups (500 mL) of broth, the spinach, jalapeño peppers, and lime zest and juice. Cook just until heated through and spinach starts to wilt. Garnish with cilantro (if using).

TIP

- If you love spicy foods, increase the number of jalapeño peppers to taste or stir in the seeds. The more seeds you add, the hotter it will be!

PER SERVING (1⅓ CUPS/325 ML) 234 calories • 2 g fat • 0 g saturated fat • 43 g carbohydrates • 10 g sugars • 10 g fibre • 10 g protein • 396 mg sodium

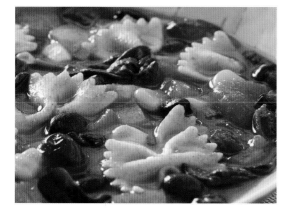

2 tsp (10 mL) extra virgin olive oil

1 small red onion, chopped

1 red bell pepper, chopped

¼ cup (60 mL) dried cranberries

4 cloves garlic, minced

1 Tbsp (15 mL) chili powder

1 tsp (5 mL) ground cumin

¾ tsp (4 mL) salt

¾ tsp (4 mL) freshly ground black pepper

8 cups (2 L) lower-sodium vegetable broth, divided

1 can (14 oz/398 mL) diced tomatoes (no salt added)

2 cans (14 oz/398 mL each) black beans (no salt added), drained and rinsed

2 cups (500 mL) whole-grain pasta bows

1 cup (250 mL) corn kernels (frozen or canned; if canned, buy unsalted and drain before using)

4 cups (1 L) loosely packed baby spinach

2 jalapeño peppers, seeded and chopped

Grated peel (zest) and juice of 1 lime

Fresh cilantro leaves, chopped (optional)

GRATITUDE—AN ESSENTIAL INGREDIENT FOR LIVING LIFE WELL

> "If the only prayer you said was thank you, that would be enough."
> **MEISTER ECKHART**

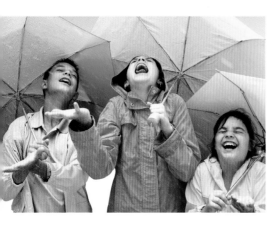

I DON'T KNOW OF one single program, teacher, or guru devoted to spirituality or self-development who doesn't teach gratitude. Not one. It is considered an absolute prerequisite to happiness and joy. To master gratitude, therefore, is truly a worthy and noble pursuit. So how does one do it? How does one become a master of something so grand? Certainly, expressing thanks to all those who cross your path each day is a start. Being aware of those less fortunate than you can also help you appreciate your blessings. A gratitude journal is yet another way to take note of the most wonderful parts of your day. I believe, however, to truly master gratitude, you must become grateful for it all. This means being grateful for the ups, the downs, and the in-betweens. It means appreciating when times are easy, but also when times are hard. It means being thankful for the joy and the laughter, but also for the heartache and the tears. It is all of these things combined that make life the masterpiece that it is. The hills and the valleys, the sunshine and the rain, sculpt us into the incredibly brave and strong human beings that we are. All of life's complexities make each moment special and allows us to learn or gain something from every situation thrown our way. Are you willing to look for the good in everything? Are you willing to say thank you for it all? Those who do, I believe, reap rewards far greater than imagined. Do your best. Life—all of life—is worth being grateful for.

LESSON LEARNED

When you say *thank you* to life—all of life—you say *thank you* to living. That's what real gratitude looks like and how a good life is lived.

Spicy Butternut Squash and Sweet Potato Soup

When my neighbour Mike tasted this soup, he said it was another "home run." I love getting home runs, especially when it comes to recipes! I hope you enjoy this as much as Mike did. It's loaded with great flavour as well as great nutrition, including beta-carotene-rich squash and sweet potatoes and fibre-rich peas. I call it a "feel good" soup. Try it and see just how good it makes you feel! **SERVES** 8

1. In a large pot over medium heat, heat the oil. Add the onions and celery and sauté until the onions are just starting to brown, about 3 minutes. Add the ginger and garlic and sauté for another 30 seconds.
2. Add the chicken broth, squash, sweet potatoes, salt, cumin, turmeric, dried red pepper flakes, and black pepper. Let simmer with the lid on for 20 to 30 minutes or until the squash and sweet potatoes are softened.
3. Add the peas and simmer for another 5 minutes.
4. Using a blender (regular or hand-held), purée the soup. Stir in the cilantro and serve immediately.

TIP

• To save time, use the pre-cubed fresh or frozen squash and sweet potato you can get at the grocery store.
• This soup is a little on the spicy side. If you are serving it to young kids, you can omit the turmeric and dried red pepper flakes (or use half the amount).

PER SERVING (1¾ CUPS/435 ML) 165 calories • 3.5 g fat •
0.5 g saturated fat • 32 g carbohydrates • 7.5 g sugars • 6 g protein •
385 mg sodium

2 Tbsp (30 mL) extra virgin olive oil

2 medium onions, diced

1 stalk celery, diced

3 Tbsp (45 mL) minced gingerroot

4 cloves garlic, minced

8 cups (2 L) lower-sodium chicken broth

1 butternut squash, peeled, seeds removed, and cubed (about 6 cups/1.5 L)

2 medium sweet potatoes, peeled and cubed (about 3 cups/750 mL)

½ tsp (2.5 mL) salt

½ tsp (2.5 mL) ground cumin

½ tsp (2.5 mL) turmeric

½ tsp (2.5 mL) dried red pepper flakes

½ tsp (2.5 mL) freshly ground black pepper

2 cups (500 mL) frozen peas

½ cup (125 mL) chopped fresh cilantro leaves

WANT A BETTER LIFE?
WRITE A BETTER STORY!

> "At any given moment you have the power to say: this is not how the story is going to end." **UNKNOWN**

EACH OF US has a set of scripts that defines what our life—our story—should or shouldn't be. We live by these scripts, usually unconsciously. These scripts have been evolving since childhood. Some of them are good. Many of them, however, greatly limit what we're capable of and how beautiful our lives can be. We carry around scripts that say we're not smart enough, beautiful enough, or good enough. We have scripts that declare we're not worthy of great love, true happiness, or real joy. Some of our scripts proclaim that to expect more is futile. Your life is a direct reflection of your scripts and your storyboards—no more, no less. If you want a different life, you need a different story. Change doesn't happen overnight. Our scripts are often deeply embedded, part of the fabric of who we are. Change requires patience, along with ongoing, daily, persistent and diligent effort. When we write a new story with new scripts, we often have to hear it many times before it takes hold. Look at your life today. Are you happy with the story it's telling? Do some of your scripts need re-writing? If so, I hope your new scripts shatter the old ones and open the door to endless possibilities. The best way to have a magnificent life story... is to write one.

LESSON LEARNED

The scripts or beliefs you've carried from childhood and beyond determine the course of your life. If you want a different life, you need a different story. When you rewrite your story, you rewrite your life. It's that simple.

Creamy Wild Mushroom Soup with Beans and Baby Spinach

This recipe comes from Sabrina Falone, an exceptional chef and recipe developer with whom I've had the pleasure of working over the last few years. This soup is proof of her exceptional talents. It's made with super-nutritious, fibre-rich beans, along with antioxidant-rich, immune-boosting mushrooms. The dehydrated mushrooms add wonderful flavour to the broth and the puréed beans give it a velvety texture. It tastes so much richer than it is. Thanks, Sabrina! **SERVES 6**

1. In a large heat-proof bowl, cover the dehydrated mushrooms with the boiling water. Set aside.
2. Meanwhile, in a large pot over medium heat, heat the canola oil. Add the onion and cook until softened, about 5 minutes. Add the cremini mushrooms and half of the salt and pepper. Cook, stirring often, until the mushrooms are browned, 5 to 7 minutes. Stir in the garlic, thyme, bay leaf, and dried red pepper flakes (if using). Pour in the wine (if using) and cook until slightly reduced, about 1 minute. Add the dehydrated mushroom and water mixture and the kidney beans, and season with the remaining salt and pepper; bring to a boil. Reduce the heat to low and simmer for about 20 minutes or until the soup is slightly thickened. Discard the thyme sprigs and bay leaf.
3. In batches, transfer the mixture to a blender and purée until very smooth (or use a hand-held blender).
4. Stir in the spinach and vinegar. Add water to reach desired consistency. Adjust the salt, pepper, and vinegar to taste. Serve and enjoy!

TIPS

- If you use beans with "no added salt," you can add another ½ tsp (2.5 mL) of salt to the soup before serving.

PER SERVING (1½ CUPS/375 ML) 248 calories • 5.4 g fat • 0.3 g saturated fat • 34 g carbohydrates • 3 g sugars • 9 g fibre • 13 g protein • 335 mg sodium

2 cups (500 mL) mixed dehydrated mushrooms, such as porcini, oyster, and portobello

6 cups (1.5 L) boiling water

2 Tbsp (30 mL) canola oil

1 onion, chopped

6 cups (1.5 L) sliced cremini mushrooms

1 tsp (5 mL) salt, divided

½ tsp (2.5 mL) freshly ground black pepper, divided

4 cloves garlic, minced

4 sprigs fresh thyme

1 bay leaf

¼ tsp (1 mL) dried red pepper flakes (optional)

½ cup (125 mL) white wine (optional)

2 cans (19 oz/540 mL each) white kidney beans, drained and rinsed

2 cups (500 mL) loosely packed baby spinach, thinly sliced

1 tsp (5 mL) white wine vinegar

BEING HELD IN SOMEONE'S ARMS IS A BEAUTIFUL PLACE TO BE

> "Millions and millions of years would still not give me half enough time to describe that tiny instant of all eternity when you put your arms around me and I put my arms around you." **JACQUES PRÉVERT**

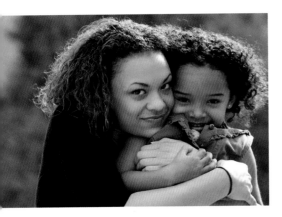

WHEN WAS THE last time you held a baby in your arms? The last time you lay in bed wrapped in the arms of someone you love? The last time you enjoyed a movie, watched the sun rise or set, sat by an ocean, or danced slowly—in someone's arms? When was the last time you comforted a child or a friend by holding them in your arms? Holding someone in your arms or being held by someone is an experience like no other. It's a beautiful place to be. It's a place of peace, calm, safety, and connection. It is a place of love. It's a place where time stands still (or you want it to). Holding someone is different than hugging someone. To hold someone is to really hold on to them—to encircle them with your arms, feel them with your heart, and not let them go. To hold someone is to heal someone and to share the magnificence of human touch. It's about sharing the beauty of the human spirit and communicating what words don't have the power to say. Is there someone special you would like to hold today? Is there someone special you would like to have hold you?

LESSON LEARNED

Few things in life are more beautiful, more healing, and more bonding than holding someone you love or having them hold you.

Spicy Red Lentil Soup

This recipe comes from Healthy Starts Here *by Mairlyn Smith, my friend and the co-author of my last two books. Mairlyn is the master of combining great taste with great nutrition. This recipe is no exception: red lentils are nutritional powerhouses and antioxidant all-stars; turmeric is king of the disease-fighting spice world; apricots are an exceptional source of beta-carotene; and tomatoes are loaded with health-protective lycopene. Thanks, Mairlyn! Enjoy!* **SERVES 4**

1. In a small bowl, combine the turmeric, cumin, cinnamon, black pepper, and allspice. Set aside.
2. Heat a large pot over medium heat. Add the oil, then the onions and celery, and sauté until golden brown, about 5 minutes.
3. Add the garlic, ginger, and the prepared spice mixture, and sauté for 1 minute.
4. Add the broth, tomatoes, lentils, apricots, and water, and bring to a boil. Reduce the heat to low and simmer, covered and stirring occasionally, until the lentils are tender, 30 to 40 minutes. Serve immediately.

TIP

• Red lentils are smaller and cook faster than their green and brown cousins. Find them with the dried beans in your local grocery store.

PER SERVING (2 CUPS/500 ML) 249 calories • 3.3 g fat • 1.4 g saturated fat • 42.9 g carbohydrates • 15.2 g sugars • 8 g fibre • 15 g protein • 465 mg sodium

1 tsp (5 mL) turmeric

1 tsp (5 mL) ground cumin

1 tsp (5 mL) ground cinnamon

1 tsp (5 mL) freshly ground black pepper

¼ tsp (1 mL) ground allspice

2 Tbsp (30 mL) extra virgin olive oil

2 onions, diced

1 cup (250 mL) chopped celery (about 3 stalks)

4 large cloves garlic, minced

1 tsp (5 mL) finely grated gingerroot

4 cups (1 L) lower-sodium chicken or vegetable broth

1 can (28 oz/796 mL) diced tomatoes

1 cup (250 mL) dried red lentils, rinsed and drained

8 dried apricots, coarsely chopped

1 cup (250 mL) water

BE RUTHLESS IN YOUR HONESTY IF YOU WANT TO BE YOUR BEST

> "Honesty is the first chapter in the book of wisdom." **THOMAS JEFFERSON**

IT'S BEEN SAID that honesty is the single most important factor in a healthy relationship. The relationship you have with yourself determines the health of all your other relationships. Therefore, if you want to master life, the person you most need to be honest with is *you*. I'm not talking about just any old honesty. I'm talking about *ruthless* honesty. I'm talking about taking off your dark sunglasses and seeing who you really are. In other words, put everything you say and do under the microscope. Ask yourself the hard questions: What do I really feel in this situation? Scared, happy, alone, guilty, angry, resentful? What do I really want in this situation? Do I want someone to like me, love me, or approve of me? Is this the best I can do in this situation? Am I making excuses for not doing more? It takes tremendous courage to be ruthlessly honest. Sometimes we don't like what we see. Sometimes we're not proud of who we are. Be kind and compassionate in your honesty. We're only human; we're not meant to be perfect. Know, however, that without honesty change is not possible. Without honesty, we will never grow and fully become who we are meant to be. Be honest. Be *ruthlessly* honest. It's the only way to truly *live*.

LESSON LEARNED

You'll never get where you want to go if you don't acknowledge where you are. Ruthless honesty is your ticket to being all you can be.

Hot Ginger Garlic Soup with Veggies and Beans

If you want a bit more zing in your life, then you should definitely try this soup. It's got great zing! It also contains two superstar vegetables—carrots and spinach—along with nutrient-rich, fibre-loaded kidney beans. It's also fast and easy to prepare. What more could you ask for? **SERVES 4**

1. In a large pot over medium heat, heat the oil. Add the onions and sauté until softened, 2 to 3 minutes. Add the ginger and garlic and sauté for another 30 seconds.
2. Add the chicken broth, beans, spinach, carrots, chili sauce, salt, and pepper. Let simmer, with the lid on, for about 5 minutes or until the carrots are tender-crisp.
3. Add the cilantro just before serving. Top with a sprinkle of freshly grated Parmesan (if using).

TIPS

- If you use beans with no added salt, you may need to add an extra ¼ tsp (1 mL) of salt. Taste first and then decide.
- Sweet chili sauce is widely available in most supermarkets and can usually be found with either the condiments or the sauces and marinades. If you don't have it on hand, you can substitute 2 tsp (10 mL) of pure maple syrup and ¼ tsp (1 mL) dried red pepper flakes.

PER SERVING (2 CUPS/500 ML) 230 calories • 4.5 g fat •
0.5 g saturated fat • 37 g carbohydrates • 5.4 g sugars • 9 g fibre •
12 g protein • 450 mg sodium

1 Tbsp (15 mL) extra virgin olive oil

1 medium onion, chopped

1 Tbsp (15 mL) minced gingerroot

3 cloves garlic, minced

4 cups (1 L) lower-sodium chicken broth

1 can (540 mL/19oz) red kidney beans, drained and rinsed

2 cups (500 mL) loosely packed baby spinach (or baby kale)

3 medium carrots, diced

1 Tbsp (15 mL) sweet chili sauce

¼ tsp (1 mL) salt

¼ tsp (1 mL) freshly ground black pepper

¼ cup (60 mL) chopped fresh cilantro leaves

Parmesan cheese (optional)

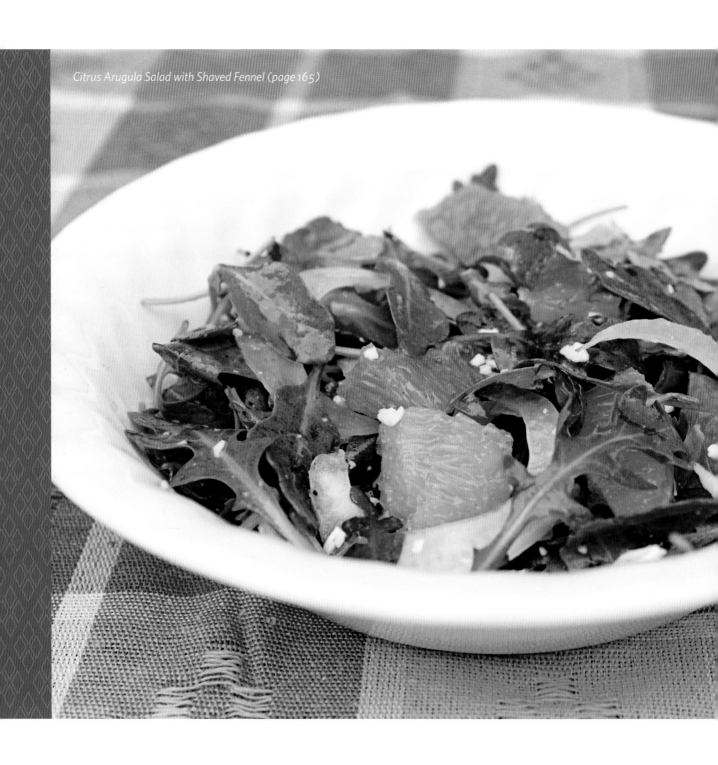
Citrus Arugula Salad with Shaved Fennel (page 165)

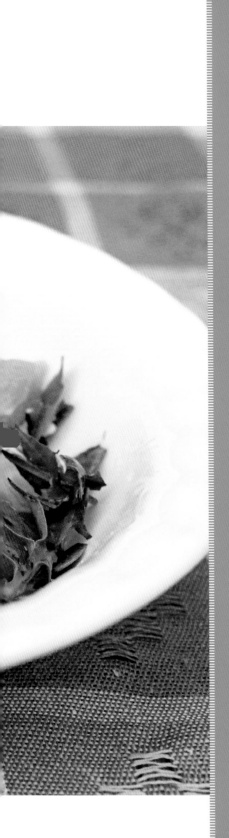

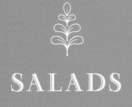

SALADS

*A life lesson comes with
every recipe. Enjoy!*

ARE YOU AN A+ STUDENT OF LIFE?

MY YOUNGEST DAUGHTER, Shannon, is a teenager. She's not an A+ student at school. She does well, sometimes very well, and sometimes not so well. I used to really care about what Shannon achieved in school. Today, I still care, but much less. Why? If someone were handing out grades for living life well, Shannon would get an A+. Shannon is a girl who cherishes her friends, loves to laugh, and loves to have fun. She lives in the moment and for the moment, happy to run in the rain or wade through a river in her bare feet. She embraces all of her emotions and feels things deeply. She's honest, open, and tells you what she thinks. Shannon rarely ends a conversation without saying "I love you." Recently I went to parent–teacher interviews. In one of the interviews, the teacher started by saying, "Sometimes Shannon gets distracted in class." He ended the interview by saying, "But you know what? I'd really love to be her." Wouldn't you?

> "The most important thing is to enjoy your life—to be happy—it's all that matters." **AUDREY HEPBURN**

LESSON LEARNED

Sometimes when we evaluate our lives and our children's lives we forget to look at the big picture. Make sure that your assessments include those things that really matter most, like happiness, love, and living life well.

Spinach Salad with Blueberries and Almonds

Would you like a totally delicious way to fit more spinach into your eating plan? Try this salad. It's one of my favourites. When I serve it to company, they always ask for more. It contains not one but three superstar ingredients: spinach, blueberries, and almonds. The dressing is fast, easy, and definitely tasty. Enjoy! **SERVES 4**

1. In a large bowl, combine all of the salad ingredients. Set aside.
2. In a small bowl, whisk together all the dressing ingredients (or put them in a small jar with a tight-fitting lid and shake well).
3. Gently toss the salad with the dressing and serve.

TIP

- Toasting the almonds is optional, but it does intensify their flavour. To toast almonds, place them in a single layer in a dry skillet over medium heat. Toast, stirring occasionally, until almonds are fragrant, 2 to 3 minutes.

PER SERVING (2½ CUPS/625 ML) 170 calories • 12 g fat • 2.5 g saturated fat • 12.5 g carbohydrates • 7.5 g sugars • 3 g fibre • 5.5 g protein • 140 mg sodium

SALAD

8 cups (2 L) loosely packed baby spinach

1 cup (250 mL) fresh blueberries

⅓ cup (80 mL) crumbled light feta cheese

¼ cup (60 mL) slivered almonds, toasted

DRESSING

1½ Tbsp (22.5 mL) extra virgin olive oil

1 Tbsp (15 mL) pure maple syrup

2 tsp (10 mL) freshly squeezed lemon juice

1 tsp (5 mL) apple cider vinegar

¼ tsp (1 mL) freshly ground black pepper

IF YOU WANT SOMETHING, GO AFTER IT

> "If you don't go after what you want, you'll never have it. If you don't ask, the answer is always no. If you don't step forward, you're always in the same place." **NORA ROBERTS**

VERY EARLY IN my career I worked for a company that did not share the same values and morals as I did. Working there was really hard for me. By the time I left, I was more than ready to go. I made a decision that the next company I worked for was going to be different. I bought a book called *100 Best Companies to Work for in Canada*. I read it cover to cover and decided that one particular company looked like the right fit for me. It was in the healthcare field and very close to home (commuting was something I didn't want to do). To get hired by this company was no easy task. They hired primarily top business grads from two of the best universities in the country. I was, however, determined. It was Christmastime. I put my carefully written resumé in a beautiful gold box with a big red bow. I addressed it to the president of the company and hand-delivered it to the main reception. Along with my resumé, I included one of my favourite quotes: "Excellence can be attained if you: Risk more than others think is safe. Care more than others think is wise. Dream more than others think is practical. Expect more than others think is possible." After multiple interviews, I got a job there. The president put the quote on a plaque on the wall of his office. Best of all, I loved working there and it was a great experience. Is there something you want in your life right now? Are you going after it?

LESSON LEARNED

Don't expect life to land in your lap. If you want something, go after it.

Baby Kale, Cranberry, and Walnut Salad

Over the last few years I've had the pleasure of working with Amy Snider-Whitson. She runs The Test Kitchen, a company that specializes in recipe development, food writing, and nutrient analysis. Amy is great at what she does, and she graciously contributed this totally delicious and definitely nutritious main-course salad. It's made with baby kale, which is milder, sweeter, and more convenient to use than traditional kale and is now widely available in the packaged lettuce section of most supermarkets. Kale is definitely a superfood your body thanks you for eating. The main source of protein in this salad is shelled edamame (soybeans not in the pod), which is also rich in fibre, potassium, and B vitamins. Edamame is available conveniently pre-shelled in the freezer section of most supermarkets. This colourful salad is great for lunch or a quick, satisfying supper after a busy day. Thanks, Amy! Enjoy! **MAKES 2 SERVINGS (DOUBLES EASILY)**

1. In a large bowl, combine all of the salad ingredients. Set aside.
2. In a small bowl, whisk together the dressing ingredients (or put them in a small jar with a tight-fitting lid and shake well).
3. Gently toss the salad with the dressing. Adjust the seasonings to taste and serve.

PER SERVING (2½ CUPS/625 ML) 420 calories • 22 g fat •
2.5 g saturated fat • 40 g carbohydrates • 24 g sugars • 10 g fibre •
15 g protein • 315 mg sodium

SALAD

4 cups (500 mL) loosely packed baby kale leaves

1 cup (250 mL) shelled edamame (thawed if frozen)

1 stalk celery, chopped

1 small carrot, grated

¼ cup (60 mL) dried cranberries

¼ cup (60 mL) walnuts, toasted and coarsely chopped

DRESSING

1 Tbsp (15 mL) cranberry or apple juice

1 Tbsp (15 mL) cider vinegar

1 Tbsp (15 mL) canola oil

2 tsp (10 mL) grainy mustard

2 tsp (10 mL) pure maple syrup

¼ tsp (1 mL) freshly ground black pepper

Pinch of salt

YOUR BODY IS WISE; LISTEN TO WHAT IT SAYS

> "There is more wisdom in your body than in your deepest philosophy."
>
> **FRIEDRICH NIETZSCHE**

MY MOTHER IS in her mid-eighties. She asked me to accompany her to an open house at a retirement home she wanted to see. During the group tour, we had to squeeze into an elevator. As I was squeezing in, I had an overwhelming sense that we should get out. I ignored it. The doors closed. They would not open and we were stuck. It was hot. There were 12 of us crammed in there and almost everyone was over the age of 80. It took two different fire departments and what seemed like forever before they finally got us out. The moral of this story? Listen to your gut. Just as animals have incredibly strong instincts, so do people. The key is to tune in to those instincts and listen to the wisdom your body has to share. Many of us, unfortunately, have learned to ignore body intelligence. Don't. You can discover so much, such as whether someone is lying or telling the truth, whether you're safe or in danger, whether you're making a good decision or a bad one. Tune in. Your body communicates loudly when you listen. It can help you live. It can save your life.

LESSON LEARNED

Never ignore your "inner voice," gut feeling, or instinct. It often tells you what you really need to know.

Citrus Arugula Salad with Shaved Fennel

My brother's daughter, Sarah (whom I love dearly!), works in a restaurant called Sorrel in Yorkville, Toronto. Sarah shared the restaurant's arugula salad recipe with me. With their permission, I played with the ingredients, including the dressing, to lighten it up a bit. Arugula is a nutrient-packed dark leafy green that's loaded with vitamin K and beta-carotene. Citrus, of course, is a vitamin C all-star, and fennel is rich in potassium as well as antioxidants. When my neighbour Elena tasted this salad, she told me I couldn't leave until I gave her the recipe. Enjoy!

P.S. This is a great recipe to serve company, too. **SERVES 4**

1. In a large bowl, combine all of the salad ingredients. Set aside.
2. In a small bowl, whisk together the dressing ingredients (or put them in a small jar with a tight-fitting lid and shake well).
3. Gently toss the salad with the dressing and serve.

TIPS
- If you're short on time, buy pre-segmented orange and grapefruit (you need about 3 cups/750 mL).
- If you're not familiar with fennel, now is a great time to get acquainted. You can find lots of videos on the internet to show you how to shave fennel if you've never done it before—a mandolin works best.

PER SERVING (2 CUPS/500 ML) 193 calories • 12 g fat •
2.5 g saturated fat • 18 g carbohydrates • 11 g sugars • 3.5 g fibre •
4 g protein • 279 mg sodium

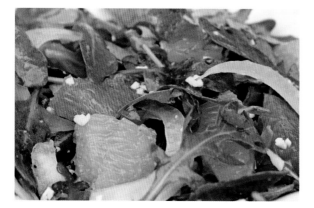

SALAD

8 cups (2 L) loosely packed arugula

1 cup (250 mL) fennel, very thinly shaved

1 large ruby red grapefruit, peeled and diced

1 navel orange, peeled and diced

⅓ cup (80 mL) crumbled light feta cheese

DRESSING

3 Tbsp (45 mL) extra virgin olive oil

2 tsp (10 mL) freshly squeezed lemon juice

1 tsp (5 mL) grated lemon peel (zest)

2 tsp (10 mL) red wine vinegar

2 tsp (10 mL) liquid honey

1 tsp (5 mL) Dijon mustard

1 green onion, chopped (white and green parts)

½ tsp (2.5 mL) freshly ground black pepper

¼ tsp (1 mL) salt

GREAT RELATIONSHIPS, INCLUDING MARRIAGES, ARE LIKE ROWING A BOAT

> "Coming together is a beginning; keeping together is progress; working together is success."
>
> **HENRY FORD**

SUCCESSFUL RELATIONSHIPS AND rowing a boat have a lot in common. First, you have to be prepared before getting into the boat. This means knowing who you are, liking who you are, and being who you are (not who you *think* you are supposed to be or who others want you to be). For most people, this step requires courage and hard work. Skip this step and your voyage may be doomed. Many people get into the boat too soon. Second, once you are ready for your trip, you need to determine your best travelling companion. Having someone who shares your core values and life philosophy is essential. If you're both well-matched intellectually and share common interests, that's a definite advantage. Having some kind of chemistry is an obvious must. Third, when you finally get into the boat, both people have to want to be there and have the same general destination in mind. Last, both people have to row! You don't always have to row at the same time, but you each have to do your part. The more you row together, the better life will be. If one person doesn't want to row, in most cases, you can't make them. You also can't make someone stay in your boat if they'd rather be in another boat. Now for the good news: If you prepare for your trip properly, have the right travelling companion, and both of you are dedicated rowers, your journey can truly be the trip of a lifetime.

LESSON LEARNED

Successful relationships require two people who know who they are and what they want. Both people have to be committed to doing the work required to make the relationship all that they want it to be.

Kale and Roasted Cauliflower Salad with Parmesan

If you don't love me yet, I think you will after you try this dish. It tastes fantastic, and it is so good for you! It contains not one but two superstar vegetables: kale and cauliflower. They are both potent cancer-fighters. Kale is especially nutrient-rich, and all the cells in your body jump up and down with joy when you eat it. The inspiration for this recipe comes from my brother's son, Aaron. Thanks, Aaron! Enjoy! **SERVES 4 TO 6**

1. Preheat the oven to 425°F (220°C).
2. In a medium bowl, whisk together the oil, lemon juice, garlic, pepper, and salt. Set aside.
3. Add the cauliflower to the oil mixture and toss to coat well.
4. Arrange the cauliflower in a single layer on a baking sheet lined with parchment paper. Roast for 25 to 30 minutes, turning halfway through. (The cauliflower should be tender-crisp when done.) As soon as it comes out of the oven, toss the hot cauliflower with the Parmesan.
5. Meanwhile, make the kale salad. Using a sharp knife, remove the thick stem that runs along the centre of each kale leaf. Chop or tear the kale leaves into bite-size pieces. (You should have about 12 cups/3L loosely packed chopped kale.) In a large bowl, whisk together the oil, lemon juice, maple syrup, salt, and pepper. Add the prepared kale. Using your hands, massage the dressing into the kale leaves until fully coated.
6. Add the roasted cauliflower to the kale salad and toss to combine well. Serve immediately.

TIPS

- Although roasted cauliflower and kale go great together, you can also enjoy either one as a standalone dish. I make this salad using just the kale all the time.
- For extra taste and nutrition, including protein, add ½ cup (125 mL) roasted pine nuts or toasted almonds.

PER SERVING (2 CUPS/500 ML) 215 calories • 10 g fat • 2 g saturated fat • 27 g carbohydrates • 4 g sugars • 7 g fibre • 11 g protein • 345 mg sodium

ROASTED CAULIFLOWER

1 Tbsp (15 mL) extra virgin olive oil

1 Tbsp (15 mL) freshly squeezed lemon juice

3 cloves garlic, minced

¼ tsp (1 mL) freshly ground black pepper

Pinch of salt

1 head cauliflower, cut into bite-size pieces (about 6 cups/1.5 L)

¼ cup (60 mL) freshly grated Parmesan cheese

SALAD

1 large bunch of kale

1 Tbsp (15 mL) extra virgin olive oil

2 tsp (10 mL) freshly squeezed lemon juice

1 tsp (5 mL) pure maple syrup

Pinch of salt

¼ tsp (1 mL) freshly ground black pepper

AMONG THE GREATEST OF ALL VIRTUES

> "Love and compassion are necessities, not luxuries. Without them humanity cannot survive."
>
> **DALAI LAMA**

TO HAVE TRUE compassion for another is to have a deep awareness and caring about the suffering of another. It is considered one of the greatest virtues. How do you develop this virtue? Certainly if you've experienced deep suffering yourself, you have a greater understanding of what it means to suffer. Compassion, however, goes far beyond just understanding. It also involves a real capacity to care. Like every other significant virtue, compassion is best achieved when it begins with you. When you sincerely embrace compassion for your own suffering, you become ready to genuinely embrace the suffering of another. How do you practise this? It's not about throwing a pity party for yourself or feeling sorry for yourself. It's about having the courage to sit deeply in your own suffering and getting to know it intimately—to look at it, to feel it, and, ultimately, to be caring about it. Can you do that for yourself? Can you do that for others?

LESSON LEARNED

Having compassion or empathy for the suffering of others is considered one of the greatest of all virtues. One of the best ways to master compassion for others is to first master compassion for yourself.

Quinoa Salad with Black Beans, Apples, and Red Grapes

How would you like a totally awesome, totally delicious, totally nutritious salad? Try this recipe. It's loaded with superstar ingredients and tastes fantastic. It's great anytime, but I highly recommend it as a take-to-work lunch. Make it on the weekend and enjoy it all week long. My eldest daughter, Chelsea, helped me create it. Thanks, Chelsea! I hope you love it as much as we do! It's so good! **SERVES 6**

1. Cook 1 cup (250 mL) of quinoa according to package directions. (One cup of uncooked quinoa makes about 3 cups/750 mL of cooked quinoa.) Cook with low-sodium chicken or vegetable broth, instead of water, for more flavour. Set aside to cool.
2. Put the chopped apples, grapes, cilantro, and black beans, in a large bowl. Add the cooked quinoa.
3. Whisk together the dressing ingredients. Pour over the salad ingredients. Mix until thoroughly combined. Enjoy immediately or put in the fridge and eat it later the same day or later in the week (keeps for about 3 to 4 days). My daughter and I enjoy it most served cold— the time spent in the fridge gives the flavours a chance to mingle and come alive!

PER SERVING (1¾ CUP/435 ML) 342 calories • 9 g fat • 1 g saturated fat • 56 g carbohydrates • 16 g sugars • 9.5 g fibre • 11 g protein • 166 mg sodium

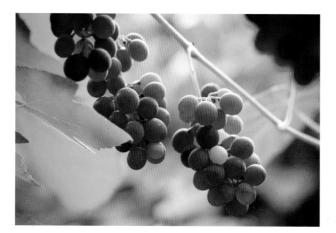

SALAD

3 cups (750 mL) cooked quinoa

2 diced Gala or Fuji apples (leave skin on)

2 cups (500 mL) red seedless grapes, halved

½ cup (125 mL) chopped fresh cilantro

1 can (19 oz/540 mL) of black beans, no salt added, drained and rinsed

DRESSING

¼ cup (60 mL) orange juice

3 Tbsp (45 mL) extra virgin olive oil

1 tsp (5 mL) freshly grated lemon peel (zest)

1 Tbsp (15 mL) fresh lemon juice

2 tsp (10 mL) pure maple syrup

2 tsp (10 mL) Dijon mustard

2 tsp (10 mL) cumin

2 tsp (10 mL) minced fresh ginger root

3 green onions, diced (including the green part)

¼ tsp (1 mL) salt

¼ tsp (1 mL) freshly ground black pepper

¼ tsp (1 mL) dried red pepper flakes (optional)

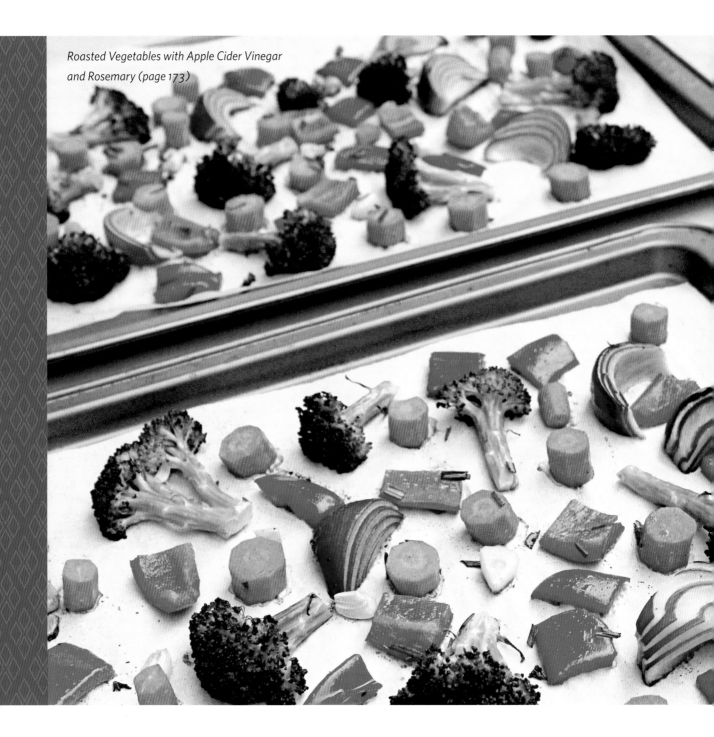

Roasted Vegetables with Apple Cider Vinegar and Rosemary (page 173)

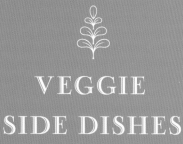

VEGGIE
SIDE DISHES

*A life lesson comes with
every recipe. Enjoy!*

WHY THE LOSS OF A PARENT IS GIANT SIZE

> "What we have once enjoyed deeply we can never lose. All that we love deeply becomes a part of us."
>
> **HELEN KELLER**

I RECENTLY ATTENDED A funeral for a man who was a significant part of my childhood. He was a farmer and his name was Johny. He lived up the road from our farm (we lived in the city, but spent every weekend and all of our summers growing up on a farm). Johny helped us cultivate our land and take care of our cows. Growing up, I spent a great deal of time at his farm and with his children. Johny lived a good, long life, and at his funeral many kind words were shared about him. After the funeral, there was a luncheon. It was here that I got to reconnect with Johny's children. I asked each of them what they loved most about their dad. Shirley, the youngest of the four kids, thought about it for a moment and then said, "What I loved most about my dad is that I knew he really loved me." Is there a more beautiful answer than that? Isn't that what parents do best? The reason losing a parent hurts so much is because the love we share with them is giant size. It's big, beautiful, and all encompassing. It can't be replaced. Whether your parents are alive or not, take some time to truly appreciate the giant-size love you share with them. There is nothing more magnificent, more incredible, and more wonderful.

LESSON LEARNED

The love we share with our parents is BIG love. It's all encompassing. Appreciate how special and how truly irreplaceable that love is and always will be.

Roasted Vegetables with Apple Cider Vinegar and Rosemary

I love roasted vegetables! So do my kids. Roasting or grilling brings out their natural sweetness. In this dish, I combine three super-nutritious all-star vegetables—broccoli, carrots, and red peppers—with onions and garlic. My daughter likes this recipe so much, she often asks me to make extra so she can pack it in her lunch the next day. Enjoy! **SERVES 4**

1 head of broccoli, cut into small trees

1 red bell pepper, diced

3 carrots, cut into coins

1 small red onion, cut into wedges

3 cloves garlic

2 Tbsp (30 mL) extra virgin olive oil

1 Tbsp (15 mL) apple cider vinegar

1 Tbsp (15 mL) dried rosemary

¼ tsp (1mL) freshly ground black pepper

Pinch of salt

1. Preheat the oven to 400°F (200°C).
2. Wash the broccoli, pepper, and carrots and pat dry (leaving too much water clinging to them will steam instead of roast the veggies). Using a sharp knife, cut the veggies and onion into similar-size pieces (the smaller you cut them, the faster they'll cook). Peel the garlic and cut it into quarters.
3. In a large bowl, whisk together the oil, vinegar, and rosemary. Add the prepared veggies and garlic, and toss until well coated.
4. Spread the seasoned vegetables in a single layer on a baking sheet lined with parchment paper (they should not be piled on top of each other). Season with pepper and, lightly, with salt. Roast for 30 to 40 minutes, stirring every 10 minutes, until vegetables are tender-crisp and just starting to turn golden brown to black. Serve immediately.

TIPS

- You can use any combination of veggies for this recipe; just make sure you have about 6 cups (1.5 L) total of cut-up raw veggies to start. Other great veggies for roasting include squash, mushrooms, Brussels sprouts, and asparagus.
- If you have a kid who is a picky eater and doesn't like all their vegetables mixed together, try making this with just one kind of vegetable, such as broccoli or carrots.
- You can substitute 3 Tbsp (45 mL) fresh rosemary for the dried rosemary, but I find dried works best in this recipe.

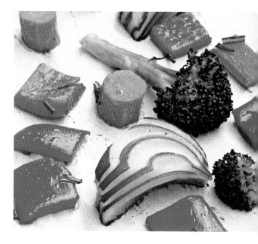

PER SERVING (1 CUP/250 ML) 105 calories • 7 g fat • 1 g saturated fat • 7 g carbohydrates • 4 g sugars • 3 g fibre • 2 g protein • 115 mg sodium

TAKING CHANCES ON THE WEST COAST TRAIL

> "Accept the challenges so that you can feel the exhilaration of victory."
>
> **GEORGE S. PATTON**

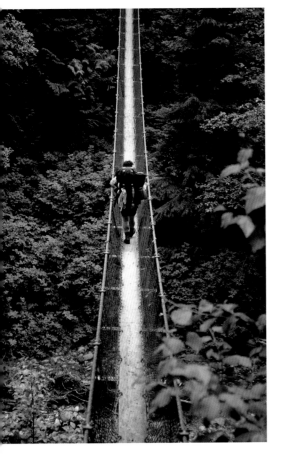

IN JULY 2011, I hiked the West Coast Trail on Vancouver Island in British Columbia. It's a 47 mile (75 km) long trail that is physically demanding and spectacularly beautiful. You carry everything on your back (40 pounds/18 kg worth of stuff), including your tent and food. This is what I learned about life and myself while hiking:

- It's great to have a big challenge on the horizon to look forward to. Training for the West Coast Trail was exciting.
- Big challenges are scary. Fear came calling the loudest my first night in the tent, before the hike even began. Could I do it? Would I make it? I really had to manage my fear. I'm glad I did. It was the hike of a lifetime. If I'd let fear win, I would have lost.
- It feels good to push myself physically. I crawled into the tent exhausted each night and fell asleep as soon as my head hit the pillow.
- I travelled with a group of people I'd never met before. Making new friends was one of the best parts of the trip, including the friends I met along the trail each day. New friends make your world bigger and brighter.
- Nature nurtures my soul like few others things can. The West Coast Trail is beautiful. Every step of the trail took my breath away. When I came home I had to adjust to living indoors again. I now prioritize spending at least some time outdoors every single day. My soul says, "thank you."

LESSON LEARNED

Big challenges are exciting and scary, but definitely worth it. You learn about yourself and about life, and experience the magnificence of what it means to be alive.

Sautéed Asparagus with Ginger and Garlic

This side dish is fast, easy, and delicious. Both adults and kids love it. I make it often—it goes great with chicken, fish, or steak. When I serve it to guests, they almost always ask for the recipe.

Asparagus is a nutrient-rich vegetable. It's an excellent source of vitamin K, a nutrient that's important for bone health and heart health and one that most people don't get enough of. It's also rich in disease-fighting folate, vitamin C, and beta-carotene. When buying asparagus, the fresher the better. Look for firm spears with closed, compact tips. Enjoy!

SERVES 4

1 bunch asparagus

1 Tbsp (15 mL) extra virgin olive oil

1 Tbsp (15 mL) minced gingerroot

2 cloves garlic, minced

⅛ tsp (0.5 mL) salt

¼ tsp (1 mL) freshly ground black pepper

2 tsp (10 mL) sugar

1. Using a sharp knife, trim the tough ends off the asparagus and cut the stalks into 1-inch (2.5 cm) pieces (you should have about 3 cups/750 mL).
2. In a large frying pan over medium heat, heat the oil. Sauté the asparagus just until tender-crisp, 3 to 5 minutes.
3. Add the ginger, garlic, salt, and pepper. Sprinkle with the sugar and sauté for about 1 minute until heated through. Serve immediately.

TIP

- If you'd prefer this a bit spicy, add ¼ tsp (1 mL) of dried red pepper flakes.

PER SERVING (¾ CUP/185 ML) 60 calories · 3.5 g fat · 0.5 g saturated fat · 6.75 g carbohydrates · 4 g sugars · 2 g fibre · 2 g protein · 75 g sodium

YOUR GREATNESS IS MAGNIFICENT... SO WHY DON'T YOU STAND IN IT?

"Every day, people settle for less than they deserve. They are only partially living or at best living a partial life. Every human being has the potential for greatness."

BO BENNETT

I BELIEVE EACH AND every one of us has greatness inside us. Not just a little bit of greatness—I'm talking brilliant, blinding, incredible, awe-inspiring, mind-blowing greatness. Rock-the-house-down greatness. I believe we are born with it, and every person's greatness is totally unique. The greatness of Mother Teresa, for example, is entirely different than the greatness of Bill Gates. How much do you stand in your greatness, your beauty? What makes you wonderful and unique? Do you stand miles away from it? Do you stand a few feet from it? Do you believe it even exists? What if I challenged you to stand right smack in the centre of your greatness? What if I dared you to claim it as yours? What would your life look like? Who would you be? Most important, what fears or limiting beliefs stop you from standing there today? We all have greatness inside us. Look for it, feel it! Give yourself permission to find it. Why? The closer you stand to your greatness, the greater your life will be.

LESSON LEARNED

True greatness lives inside all of us. Have the courage to find yours and stand in it.

Sweet Potato Fries with Allspice and Lemon Zest

Sweet potatoes are a goldmine of nutrition. They're loaded with health-protective beta-carotene as well as sought-after nutrients like vitamin C, potassium, and fibre. Over the years, I've tried lots of different recipes for sweet potatoes. This one is one of my favourites. The lemon zest, allspice, and sweet potato combination just seems like the perfect marriage of flavours. Enjoy! **SERVES 2 TO 4**

1. Preheat the oven to 400°F (200°C).
2. In a large bowl, whisk together the oil, lemon zest, allspice, pepper, and salt. Add the sweet potatoes and toss to coat well.
3. Spread the fries in a single layer on a large baking sheet lined with parchment paper.
4. Bake for 30 to 40 minutes, until tender-crisp and nicely browned, turning once halfway through the cooking time.

PER SERVING (1 CUP/250 ML) 115 calories • 3.5 g fat • 0.5 g saturated fat • 20 g carbohydrates • 6.5 g sugars • 3 g fibre • 1.6 g protein • 175 mg sodium

1 Tbsp (15 mL) extra virgin olive oil

1 tsp (5 mL) freshly grated lemon peel (zest)

½ tsp (2.5 mL) ground allspice

¼ tsp (1 mL) freshly ground black pepper

¼ tsp (1 mL) salt

2 to 3 sweet potatoes, peeled and sliced into fries (about 4 cups/1 L)

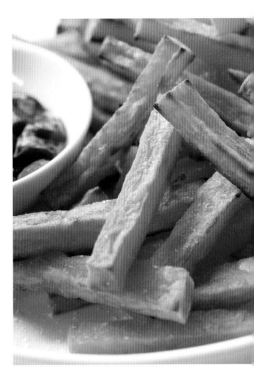

THE POWER OF AN APOLOGY

> "In some families, *please* is described as the magic word. In our house, however, it was *sorry*."
>
> **MARGARET LAURENCE**

NEVER UNDERESTIMATE THE power of a heartfelt apology. When you apologize to someone, you acknowledge their pain. When you acknowledge their pain, you give them permission to let that pain go. Letting go of pain opens the door to joy and happiness. If joy and happiness are what you want, the most important person you can say "I'm sorry" to is often yourself. Why? You can't control other people. You can't make them apologize for something they've done that feels hurtful. They may not even be aware an apology is required. They may not be capable of an apology. *You* are capable. Give it to yourself. Feel your pain fully, listen to what it has to say, then respond with the sorry that you need to hear: I'm sorry that this happened. I'm sorry it was so hard. I'm sorry you had to go through this. I'm sorry you didn't get what you wanted or needed or deserved. Say sorry and say it often. All pain, especially big pain, wants to be heard and acknowledged in its entirety before it says goodbye. Give your pain the recognition it deserves so that it knows its job is done.

LESSON LEARNED

When you listen to, acknowledge, and have true compassion for your own pain, you give yourself permission to let that pain go.

Roasted Balsamic Potatoes with Dijon and Fresh Thyme

My neighbour Mike, an amazing cook, loves potatoes and cooks them often. His wife said that if Mike likes this recipe, then it has to be good. Mike not only likes the recipe, he loves it! I use Yukon Gold potatoes, but you can also use regular white potatoes or baby potatoes. Be sure to leave the skin on for the extra nutrients and fibre. Enjoy! **SERVES 4 TO 6**

1. Preheat the oven to 400°F (200°C).
2. In a large bowl, whisk together the dressing ingredients.
3. Add the diced potatoes and toss until well coated.
4. Arrange the potatoes in a single layer on a baking sheet lined with parchment paper (be careful not to overcrowd them). Bake, turning the potatoes every 15 minutes, for 40 to 45 minutes or until tender and golden brown.

TIP
- You can also make this dish with sweet potatoes, which are higher in beta-carotene and have a lower glycemic index.

PER SERVING (1 CUP/250 ML) 152 calories · 3 g fat · 0.4 g saturated fat · 31 g carbohydrates · 4 g sugars · 4 g fibre · 3 g protein · 176 mg sodium

DRESSING

3 Tbsp (45 mL) balsamic vinegar

2 Tbsp (30 mL) fresh thyme leaves

1 Tbsp (15 mL) extra virgin olive oil

1 Tbsp (15 mL) Dijon mustard

¼ tsp (1 mL) salt

¼ tsp (1 mL) freshly ground black pepper

2 cloves garlic, minced

1 jalapeño pepper, minced

POTATOES

5 medium potatoes, skin on, diced (about 5 cups/1.25 L)

THERE IS NO REWIND BUTTON

> "Twenty years from now you will be more disappointed by the things that you didn't do than by the ones you did do. So throw off the bowlines. Sail away from the safe harbor. Catch the trade winds in your sails. Explore. Dream. Discover." **MARK TWAIN**

I F YOU COULD go back and live your life over, would you want to? Do you think you would do it better the next time around? What would you do differently? Think about it. I believe most of us, given a second chance, would do more, love more, risk more, and really live more. We'd also let a lot more things go. Newsflash: There is no rewind button on life! This is it. You can learn from yesterday, but you can't get yesterday back. You can plan for tomorrow, but it's not here yet. This day, this minute, this second is all you've got. Waste it and it's gone. Understanding and appreciating this concept is essential to a good life. How do you want to live your life? What do you want to do? Who do you want to do it with? Who do you want to be? Why not go do these things today?

LESSON LEARNED

There is no rewind button on life. You can't go back. You can't repeat it. Do your best to live a wonderful life the first time through.

Roasted Sweet Potatoes with Apples, Raisins, and Red Onion

Sweet potatoes are a nutritional goldmine and especially rich in beta-carotene. They pair perfectly with sweet spices like cinnamon and cloves. Enjoy this dish any day of the week, but consider serving it the next time you entertain guests. These potatoes go particularly well with grilled chicken or a mild white fish, such as tilapia. **SERVES 4**

1. Preheat the oven to 400°F (200°C).
2. In a large bowl, whisk together the orange juice, oil, cinnamon, cloves, and salt. Add the potatoes, apples, onion, and the raisins or currants. Mix until fully combined.
3. Spread the sweet potato mixture in a single layer on a baking sheet lined with parchment paper. Bake, turning once halfway through the baking time, for 25 to 35 minutes or until the sweet potato is cooked and slightly crisp. Serve immediately.

PER SERVING (1 CUP/250 ML) 200 calories · 3.5 g fat · 0.5 g saturated fat · 41 g carbohydrates · 20 g sugars · 6 g fibre · 183 mg sodium

¼ cup (60 mL) orange juice

1 Tbsp (15 mL) extra virgin olive oil

1 tsp (5 mL) ground cinnamon

½ tsp (2.5 mL) ground cloves

¼ tsp (1 mL) salt

2 medium sweet potatoes, peeled and diced (about 4 cups/1 L)

1 Granny Smith apple, diced (leave skin on)

1 medium red onion, sliced

¼ cup (60 mL) raisins or currants

IF YOU WANT YOUR LIFE TO BE GOOD, NOTICE WHAT FEELS GOOD

> "When I do good, I feel good. When I do bad, I feel bad. That's my religion." **ABRAHAM LINCOLN**

IF YOU WANT a compass for living life well … you've already got one. It's called "notice how it feels." Don't underestimate the power of this internal compass. When you tune in to it, it's an incredible guide. It teaches you how to live life well. The key is to pay attention to what it has to tell you. For example:

- Notice how it feels to be loving and kind as opposed to being uncaring or unkind.
- Notice how it feels to let others live their own lives rather than trying to control what others do.
- Notice how it feels to spend time with people who really love you as opposed to spending time with people who don't.
- Notice how it feels to focus on what is good in your life versus getting caught up in what's lacking.
- Notice how it feels to carry around anger, hurt, or resentment and also how it feels to let those things go.
- Notice how it feels to be open and honest rather than being secretive or dishonest.
- Notice how it feels to give your best effort versus going through the motions or not trying very hard.

The truth is that when you really start paying attention to what feels good, you start doing good, and, as a result, life gets good.

LESSON LEARNED

Notice how what you do makes you feel. Doing good generally feels good. Let this powerful internal compass teach you how to live life well.

Sautéed Spiced Carrots with Balsamic and Maple

Carrots are a nutrient-rich, disease-fighting, superstar vegetable. Similar to other orange vegetables, they're especially rich in beta-carotene. In a 10-year study from the Netherlands involving over 40,000 men and women, carrots were the vegetable most linked to a lower risk of heart disease. Other studies link carrots to a lower risk of cancer. Enjoy this vegetable side dish with chicken or fish. You can also mix these spiced carrots into cooked quinoa or brown rice. **SERVES 4**

1. In a large skillet or frying pan over medium heat, heat the oil. Add the carrots and sauté just until tender-crisp, about 5 minutes.
2. Add the vinegar, maple syrup, ginger, cinnamon, and chili powder. Sauté for about 1 minute more. Serve immediately.

PER SERVING (1 CUP/250 ML) 100 calories • 4 g fat • 0.5 g saturated fat • 17 g carbohydrates • 10 g sugars • 4 g fibre • 1 g protein • 88 mg sodium

1 Tbsp (15 mL) extra virgin olive oil

4 cups (1 L) sliced carrots (cut into coins; about 8 to 10 medium carrots)

1 Tbsp (15 mL) balsamic vinegar

1 Tbsp (15 mL) pure maple syrup

2 tsp (10 mL) minced gingerroot

½ tsp (2.5 mL) ground cinnamon

½ tsp (2.5 mL) chili powder

LIVING LIFE ON THE EXTREME EDGE

> "Life can be like a roller coaster... and just when you think you've had enough, and you are ready to get off the ride and take the calm, easy merry-go-round... you change your mind, throw your hands in the air, and ride the roller coaster all over again. That's exhilaration... that's living a bit on the edge... that's being ALIVE." **STACEY CHARTER**

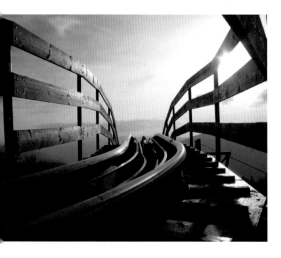

WHEN WAS THE last time you did something totally crazy—almost insane—and completely out of your comfort zone? If you can't remember then perhaps you need to get creative. Life is short! Are you here for a boring, predictable ride or do you want to throw caution to the wind, at least once in a while? Standing on the edge of life is scary, but it's also so incredibly energizing. It's like getting a shot of pure adrenaline—a shot of pure life! Do you want to feel vibrant and alive? If so, what crazy, totally insane thing would you love to do? Parachute out of a plane? Go motocrossing? Pack your bags for an unplanned weekend trip for two? Ask someone out on a date (if you're single, that is)? Remember: Your edge and someone else's edge may be totally different. Tune in to what feels scary but still exhilarating—then go for it and let me know how it works out. My guess is you'll tell me how alive and wonderful you feel and how you can't wait to do something at least a little wild and crazy again sometime soon. Life is here to be lived. Go live it!

LESSON LEARNED

Life shouldn't be boring and predictable. Do things that make you feel scared and uncomfortable. That's called living and it's what life is for!

Corn, Carrots, and Peppers with Herbs and Garlic

This is a great vegetable side dish to serve anytime, but especially at your next family gathering. It's colourful, tasty, and loved by adults and kids alike. It's also loaded with good nutrition. Corn is a fibre all-star and definitely good for gut health. It's also rich in antioxidants, including lutein and zeaxanthin, which are good for your eyes. Carrots are an exceptional source of health-protective beta-carotene. Red peppers are nutrient-rich and an outstanding source of vitamin C. The inspiration for this recipe comes from Teri Boothe. Thanks, Teri!

P.S. You don't need a crowd to make this dish—it's great for leftovers. You can make it early in the week and enjoy it all week long. I do.

SERVES 8

4 tsp (20 mL) extra virgin olive oil

4 medium carrots, very thinly sliced

1 large red bell pepper, diced

1 large jalapeño pepper (seeds removed), finely diced

2 cloves garlic, minced

1 tsp (5 mL) dried oregano leaves

1 tsp (5 mL) dried marjoram

5½ cups (1.4 L) frozen corn

½ cup (125 mL) chopped fresh basil leaves

1. In a large frying pan or skillet, preferably with a lid, heat the oil over medium heat. Add the carrots, red pepper, and jalapeño and sauté for about 2 to 3 minutes (red peppers and carrots should just be starting to soften). Add the garlic, oregano, and marjoram. Stir-fry for another 30 seconds, stirring frequently.

2. Add the corn and basil and mix until combined. Cover with a lid and cook, stirring frequently, until the corn is cooked through, 3 to 4 minutes. Serve immediately.

TIPS

- If marjoram is not something you currently have in your cupboard, be sure to buy it next time you're grocery shopping. It is a sweet-tasting herb used extensively in Mediterranean cuisine and an important addition to this dish.
- Use this veggie side dish to dress up cooked quinoa or brown rice.

PER SERVING (¾ CUP/185 ML) 130 calories · 3 g fat · 0.5 g saturated fat · 24 g carbohydrates · 5 g sugars · 4 g fibre · 4 g protein · 27 mg sodium

A MARRIAGE BUILT TO LAST

> "The best proof of love is trust."
>
> **JOYCE BROTHERS**

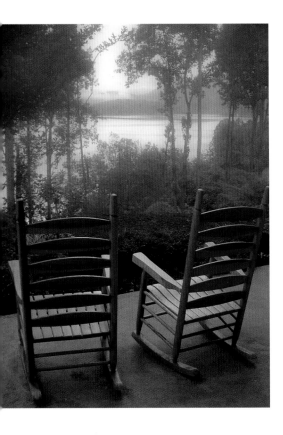

I WAS WALKING WITH one of my dearest and closest friends, Laureen, near her house. Half way through our walk it started to rain. "Don't worry, Stuart will come and get us," said Laureen. Within minutes her husband arrived in his car to pick us up. She had not called him or asked him to come. She just knew that he would. Laureen and Stuart have one of the most beautiful marriages I've ever had the honour to observe. They really love each other. They were recently voted "the couple most likely to stay together" at a neighbourhood party. I asked Laureen what she thought makes their marriage so special. "I trust Stuart with my life," she replied. How's that for an answer? But what does it mean? Laureen feels that Stuart has her back not just some of the time, but *all* of the time. She can depend on him, count on him, and not just for the little things in life, but for the really big things, too. This is a marriage based on love and built on trust. Is there a stronger foundation than that? I don't think so.

LESSON LEARNED

A marriage based on love and built on trust is a marriage made to last.

Maple-Baked Squash with Olive Oil and Fresh Thyme

Want to know a great habit to get into? Eat a vegetable that is deep orange in colour—such as squash, carrots, and sweet potatoes—every single day! These vegetables are an exceptional source of nutrients that your body needs for good health, including beta-carotene, which is linked to a lower risk of heart disease and cancer. This baked squash recipe is a healthier version of a classic favourite. Enjoy! **SERVES 4**

2 acorn squash, cut in half (seeds removed)

2 tsp (10 mL) extra virgin olive oil, divided

2 tsp (10 mL) pure maple syrup, divided

2 tsp (10 mL) chopped fresh thyme leaves, divided

¼ tsp (1 mL) freshly ground black pepper

1. Preheat the oven to 375°F (190°C).
2. Using a small, sharp knife, cut a crisscross pattern into the flesh of the squash. Be careful not to pierce the skin.
3. Place the squash, cut-side up, onto a baking sheet lined with parchment paper.
4. In a small bowl, whisk together the oil, maple syrup, thyme, and pepper. Brush evenly over the flesh of the squash.
5. Bake for about 45 minutes or until the squash is soft and pierces easily with a fork. Remove from the oven and spoon any sauce that has not been absorbed by the squash evenly over the flesh. Let cool for 5 to 10 minutes before serving.

TIPS
*   If you don't have fresh thyme, use ½ tsp (2.5 mL) dried thyme.
*   For something different, you can replace the thyme with a light sprinkle of cinnamon or nutmeg. Kids often like it this way.

PER HALF SQUASH 115 calories • 2.5 g fat • 0.4 g saturated fat • 24 g carbohydrates • 10 g sugars • 3.3 g protein • 6 g sodium

IF GROWING UP WERE EASY, I'D BE GROWN UP BY NOW

> "It takes courage to grow up and become who you really are."
>
> **E. E. CUMMINGS**

THERE ARE MANY wonderful things about being a kid: Life is carefree and easy. You don't have to think about anyone but yourself. Other people take care of you. You can cry when you don't get your way. No wonder it's so hard to grow up! Many of us would like to remain kids for our whole lives . . . and some of us do. We even believe we win by staying a kid, but ultimately we lose. We lose the opportunity to stand in our power and be all that we are capable of being. We depend on others to take care of us and lose the opportunity to take care of ourselves. We lose the opportunity to respond rather than react in any given situation and to take full responsibility for the choices we make. Each day presents endless moments when you can choose to be either a kid or an adult. I say have fun and enjoy life, but have the courage and strength to grow into the person you were meant to be.

LESSON LEARNED

Growing up is hard, but when you refuse to grow up, your life stays as small as you do.

Grilled Balsamic Broccoli

Broccoli is a cancer-fighting all-star and a nutritional powerhouse. Having fast and easy ways to fit more of it into your eating plan is important. I included this recipe because it's super fast and easy, and because most people don't think to throw broccoli on the grill. Yet broccoli on the grill is totally awesome! Both my daughters love it this way. Enjoy!

SERVES 2 TO 4

1. Preheat the grill to medium heat.
2. In a bowl, whisk together the oil, vinegar, and pepper. Add the broccoli and toss until well coated.
3. Spray the grill with non-stick vegetable oil. Arrange the broccoli in a single layer and cook for 2 to 3 minutes. Turn and grill for another 2 to 3 minutes or until the broccoli is tender-crisp. If desired, serve lightly sprinkled with freshly grated Parmesan.

TIPS

- The smaller the broccoli trees, the faster they will cook.
- This combination of olive oil and balsamic vinegar can be used to grill all kinds of vegetables, including carrots, mushrooms, peppers, onions, and asparagus. Feel free to throw some fresh herbs and minced garlic into the mixture, too.
- If you want to spice things up, add ¼ tsp (1 mL) of dried red pepper flakes.

PER SERVING (1¼ CUP/310 ML EACH) 100 calories · 7 g fat · 1 g saturated fat · 8 g carbohydrates · 2 g sugars · 3 g fibre · 3 g protein · 37 mg sodium

1 Tbsp (15 mL) extra virgin olive oil

1 tsp (5 mL) balsamic vinegar

¼ tsp (1 mL) freshly ground black pepper

1 large head broccoli, chopped into trees (about 2½ cups/ 625 mL)

Freshly grated Parmesan cheese (optional)

ONCE YOU MASTER THIS, YOU CAN MASTER ANYTHING

> "Always do what you are afraid to do." **RALPH WALDO EMERSON**

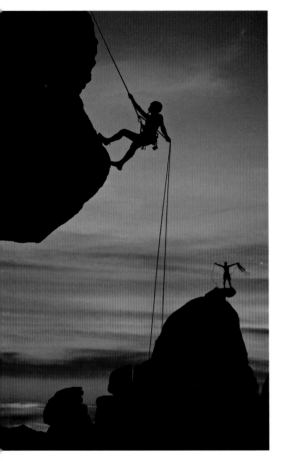

WHAT STOPS YOU from living your dream life? What holds you back from loving people with your whole heart? What prevents you from trying something totally new or completely different? The universal answer is fear. If you want to master life, you have to master fear. One of the best ways to do this is by standing right smack in the centre of it. Most people run away from fear as soon as they feel it. It's a natural human reaction and how we protect ourselves. This is the part we need to work on. How? First, become an expert at noticing when fear arrives. Second, as soon as you feel it, decide that you won't run, you won't shut down, and you will not build a fortress. Instead, stand there, right in the middle of it, and breathe. This is the hard part. Fear often hits us like a giant wave, and it feels as if we will not survive, especially when faced with our big fears. In reality, however, survival is not only possible, but likely! Have courage. Keep standing. Keep breathing. When you learn to stay with fear, rather than run from it, there's almost nothing you can't do.

LESSON LEARNED

When you don't run from fear, fear doesn't run you.

Sautéed Kale with Lemon, Maple, and Garlic

Kale has been called one of the healthiest vegetables in the world, and for good reason: Not only does it contain plant compounds that fight cancer, but it also has more nutrition per bite than most any other vegetable. It's especially rich in superstar nutrients like vitamin K, beta-carotene, and vitamin C. You can add chopped kale to soups, omelettes, quiche, rice, stir-fries, lasagna, quesadillas, or even pizza. One of the easiest ways to enjoy it, however, is simply sautéed and served as a side dish to your main meal. **SERVES 2**

½ bunch kale, chopped (about 5 cups/1.25 L, loosely packed)

2 tsp (10 mL) extra virgin olive oil

1 tsp (5 mL) freshly squeezed lemon juice

1 tsp (5 mL) pure maple syrup

1 clove garlic, minced

Pinch of dried red pepper flakes (optional)

⅛ tsp (0.5 mL) salt or less, to taste

Freshly ground black pepper, to taste

1. Using a sharp knife, remove the thick rib that runs along the centre of each kale leaf and chop the leaves into bite-size pieces. Transfer the chopped kale to a colander or salad spinner, rinse well, and spin or pat dry.
2. Heat a large skillet over medium heat. Add the oil, lemon juice, maple syrup, garlic, and red pepper flakes (if using). Cook for 30 seconds, stirring constantly.
3. Add the kale, salt, and pepper. Sauté until the leaves are tender-crisp, 3 to 5 minutes. Serve immediately.

TIP

• To save on prep time, use baby kale instead.

PER SERVING (1½ CUPS/375 ML) 135 calories • 6 g fat • 1 g saturated fat • 20 g carbohydrates • 2 g sugar • 3.5 g fibre • 5.5 g protein • 218 mg sodium

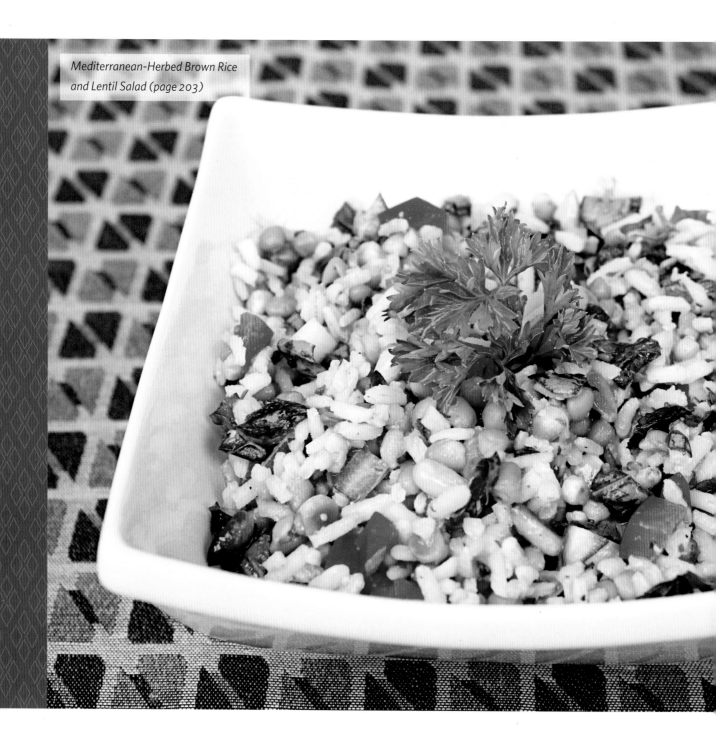

Mediterranean-Herbed Brown Rice and Lentil Salad (page 203)

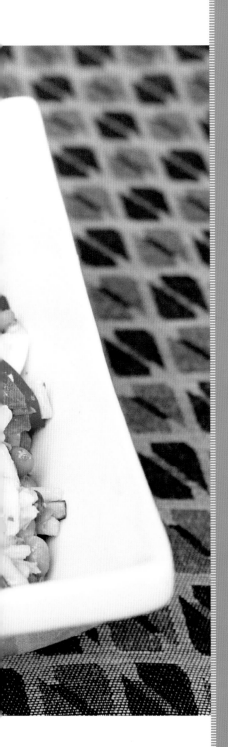

WHOLE GRAINS: PASTA, BARLEY, RICE, AND QUINOA

*A life lesson comes with
every recipe. Enjoy!*

A MASTER AT WORK IS A BEAUTIFUL THING

> "Only one who devotes himself to a cause with his whole strength and soul can be a true master. For this reason mastery demands all of a person." **ALBERT EINSTEIN**

HAVE YOU EVER had the honour of seeing a true master at work? Recently a girlfriend of mine invited me to see a fiddle rock band. The name of the band, quite appropriately, was Fiddlestix, and the lead was a guy named Steve Bowen. He plays the electric violin. I had no expectation of what the band would sound like prior to entering the bar; however, as soon as Steve started playing, I knew I was in the presence of a master. I knew that I was witnessing something extraordinary, something truly special. This was not a time to take for granted, but one to truly revel in. This guy could play the violin like no one I had ever seen before. He played fast, slow, soft, and hard. It was magical. When the band took a break, I approached Steve and asked him how long he'd been playing. He told me 38 years! He'd been playing the violin since the age of 4. I was in the presence of a master. When was the last time you saw a master at work? Was it an athlete, an artist, a speaker, a musician, a mother? Do you realize what it truly takes to be a master—the time, the passion, the dedication, the incredible heart and soul? Are you a master of something? Do you appreciate those who are?

LESSON LEARNED

There are masters in all walks of life. They put their heart and soul into learning, practising, and perfecting their craft. If you ever have the privilege to share time with one, realize what an honour it is.

Totally Terrific
Tex-Mex Bow-Tie Pasta

Here's a totally delicious way to get more whole grains, beans, and fibre into your eating plan—something most of us could use more of! It can be served hot or enjoyed as a cold pasta salad. The leftovers are great for lunch the next day. The jalapeño peppers, garlic, and chili powder give it a real flavour kick, yet it's not too hot for kids. I helped to develop this recipe while working on a campaign with Catelli Healthy Harvest® Whole-grain Pasta. I hope you love it as much as I do. Enjoy! **MAKES 6 SERVINGS**

1. In a large pot of boiling water, cook the pasta according to the package instructions.
2. Meanwhile, in a large frying pan or deep skillet over medium heat, heat the oil. Add the onion, red pepper, and jalapeños, and sauté until the onion is translucent and the red pepper is tender-crisp, 3 to 5 minutes. Add the garlic and sauté for another 30 seconds.
3. Add the black beans, corn (including all the liquid), chili powder, cumin, lemon zest, and salt. Continue cooking, stirring often, just until all the ingredients are heated through, 3 to 5 minutes. Add the vinegar and tomatoes and cook, stirring gently, for about 1 minute more or until the tomato is just heated through. Remove from the heat.
4. Transfer the black bean mixture to a large bowl and toss with the cooked pasta and the parsley. Serve immediately or cover and refrigerate to enjoy later as a cold salad.

PER SERVING (2 CUPS/500 ML) 380 calories • 7 g fat • 1 g saturated fat • 66 g carbohydrates • 6 g sugars • 12 g fibre • 16 g protein • 210 mg sodium

6 cups (1.5 L) uncooked whole-wheat pasta bows

2 Tbsp (30 mL) extra virgin olive oil

1 medium red onion, diced

1 medium red bell pepper, diced

2 jalapeño peppers, seeds removed and finely diced

3 cloves garlic, minced

1 can (19 oz/540 mL) black beans (no salt added), drained and rinsed

1 can (12 oz/355 mL) corn (no salt added)

1 Tbsp (15 mL) chili powder

1 tsp (5 mL) ground cumin

Grated peel (zest) of 1 large lemon

½ tsp (2.5 mL) salt

¼ cup (60 mL) apple cider vinegar

1 cup (250 mL) diced sweet cocktail tomatoes

1 cup (250 mL) loosely packed chopped fresh parsley leaves

LISTEN WITH GENEROSITY

> "The most basic and powerful way to connect to another person is to listen. Just listen. Perhaps the most important thing we ever give each other is our attention... A loving silence often has far more power to heal and to connect than the most well-intentioned words."
>
> **RACHEL NAOMI REMEN**

I REMEMBER MANY WONDERFUL things about growing up with my dad. Perhaps the most significant was his incredible ability to listen. He always listened with such intent, as if what I had to say really mattered. He also asked questions, always probed deeper for a better understanding of who I was and what it was I was really trying to communicate. Because of this, not only did I feel listened to, I truly felt heard and understood. I felt that what I had to say mattered and, even more importantly, that I mattered. To know that we matter is one of the most basic yet significant desires of all human beings. Each one of us wants to matter to someone. Do you make people feel they matter? Do you do your best to listen, hear, and understand what they think and feel? Never underestimate the power of doing so. Never underestimate the gift someone gives when they do this for you.

LESSON LEARNED

To be listened to, heard, and understood is perhaps the greatest gift we can receive and give. Be generous with this gift, especially with those you love. Be grateful for those who share this gift with you. This is love in one of its purest forms.

Rotini with Grape Tomatoes, Portobello Mushrooms, and Asparagus

Loaded with colourful, fresh-tasting, nutritious ingredients, this dish can be enjoyed any time: it's perfect for Sunday brunch, weekday lunch, or dinner with friends. It also tastes great warmed up or served cold the next day. Enjoy! **SERVES 6**

1. In a large pot of boiling water, cook the pasta according to the package instructions.
2. Meanwhile, in a small bowl, combine the grape tomatoes, basil, and 2 Tbsp (30 mL) of the oil. Set aside.
3. In a large frying pan over medium heat, add ¼ cup (60 mL) of the oil and the onion and sauté until onion is translucent, about 3 minutes. Add the mushrooms, asparagus, almonds, salt, pepper, and red pepper flakes and sauté for another 6 minutes or until the asparagus is tender-crisp. Add the minced ginger and garlic and sauté for another 30 seconds.
4. In a large bowl, combine the drained, cooked pasta with the sautéed vegetables. Serve with freshly grated Parmesan cheese.

PER SERVING (2 CUPS/500 ML) 462 calories • 23 g fat •
2.5 g saturated fat • 55 g carbohydrates • 3 g sugars • 10 g fibre •
17 g protein •

5 cups (1.2 L) whole-wheat rotini pasta

2 cups (500 mL) grape tomatoes, cut into halves

½ cup (125 mL) chopped fresh basil leaves

6 tablespoons (90 mL) extra virgin olive oil, divided

1 medium onion, diced

3 large portobello mushrooms, chopped (about 2 cups/ 500 mL)

1 bunch asparagus, chopped (about 3 cups/750 mL)

1 cup (250 mL) raw unsalted sliced or chopped almonds, skin on

½ tsp (2.5 mL) salt (optional)

½ tsp (2.5 mL) freshly ground black pepper

¼ tsp (1 mL) dried red pepper flakes

4 cloves garlic, minced

1 Tbsp (15 mL) minced gingerroot

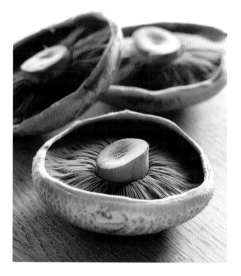

A PICNIC IS A BEAUTIFUL THING

> "I don't know why, but the meals we have on picnics always taste so much nicer than the ones we have indoors." **ENID BLYTON**

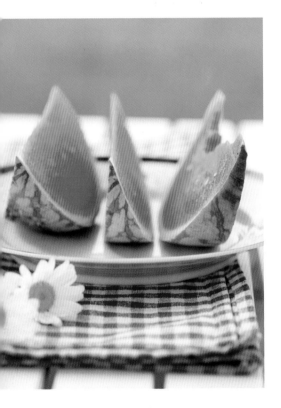

IT WAS MOTHER'S Day. I told all the moms on my street to meet me on my driveway at noon and bring lots of great food—it was time for a picnic. I have an enthusiastic group on my street, so everyone was game. We loaded up my super-big backpack with lots of yummy food and then all of us, along with our kids and one dog, hiked along the river in the ravine by our street. We hiked for about an hour, having fun along the way, and stopped at the perfect spot for a picnic. And what a picnic it was! We had wine, cheese, crackers, salads, cold chicken, shrimp, and desserts. The moms loved it. The kids loved it. The dog loved it. Weather permitting, my guess is that this picnic will become a regular Mother's Day event. Looking back on my life, I've come to realize that many of my fondest memories are from the days I experienced the joys of a picnic. There's something so exceptional about sharing a great meal with family or friends outside, in a forest, by a river, at a park, or on top of a mountain. Most people don't do it often enough. I've decided to make room for more picnics in my life. And you? When will you plan your next picnic?

LESSON LEARNED

Make room for more picnics in your life. It's a wonderful way to create awesome memories and share delicious food with family and friends in the beautiful outdoors.

Rotini Pasta Salad with Honey Ginger Mixed Greens

I helped develop this cold pasta salad recipe while working on a campaign with Catelli Healthy Harvest® Whole-grain Pasta. It's colourful and full of flavour—and easy enough to enjoy any day of the week (definitely great to serve to guests, too). It's also a wonderful dish to bring on a picnic. In fact, I suggest you plan a picnic just so you can bring this salad! The dark leafy greens combined with the vitamin E–rich almonds and sunflower seeds make it super nutritious. Enjoy! **SERVES 4**

1. Cook the rotini in boiling water according to the package instructions. Drain and rinse under cold running water. Set aside.
2. Meanwhile, place the dried fruit in a heat-proof bowl and cover with boiling water. Let stand for 5 minutes. Drain well and set aside.
3. In a small bowl, whisk together the dressing ingredients (or put them in a small jar with a tight-fitting lid and shake well).
4. In a large bowl, combine the cooked rotini with the dried fruit, leafy greens, almonds, and sunflower seeds. Add the dressing and toss to coat. Serve immediately or cover and refrigerate until serving time.

TIPS

- For extra flavour and nutrition, use a salad blend that includes fresh herbs as well as leafy greens.
- If making this dish ahead, hold back a little of the dressing to toss with the salad and moisten it at serving time.

PER SERVING (1¾ CUPS/435 ML) 444 calories • 20 g fat •
2.5 g saturated fat • 61 g carbohydrates • 14 g sugars • 8 g fibre •
10 g protein • 205 mg sodium

SALAD

3 cups (750 mL) whole-wheat rotini pasta

½ cup (125 mL) assorted dried fruit (such as cranberries, blueberries, raisins, and currants)

4 cups (1 L) lightly packed mixed baby leafy greens

¼ cup (60 mL) slivered almonds, toasted

¼ cup (60 mL) unsalted roasted sunflower seeds

DRESSING

¼ cup (60 mL) extra virgin olive oil

3 Tbsp (45 mL) orange juice

2 Tbsp (30 mL) white wine vinegar

2 Tbsp (30 mL) very finely chopped shallot

1 Tbsp (15 mL) minced gingerroot

1 Tbsp (15 mL) liquid honey

1 tsp (5 mL) finely grated orange peel (zest)

1 tsp (5 mL) Dijon mustard

1 small clove garlic, minced

¼ tsp (1 mL) salt

¼ tsp (1 mL) freshly ground black pepper

THE LANGUAGE OF THE SOUL

> "We should consider every day lost on which we have not danced at least once." **FRIEDRICH NIETZSCHE**

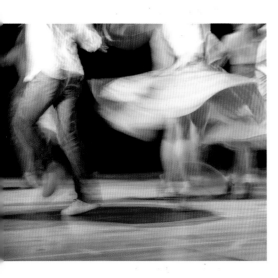

I'VE BEEN DESCRIBED as a person who never lets a good dance song go to waste. Recently I attended a wedding. It was a lovely wedding with a beautiful bride and a handsome groom. The food was great, the people I met were wonderful, but best of all was the dancing. It started at about 9 p.m. and ended at about 1:30 a.m. I danced all night! I danced with anyone and everyone—men, women, couples, singles, groups, kids, and grandparents. If they were dancing, I danced with them. As I was leaving, an elderly man tapped me on the shoulder and said, "You looked like you had the best time tonight." I did have the best time. I went home with blisters on my feet and a huge smile on my face. Dancing has been called the hidden language of the soul. Is it the language of your soul? Does it express who you are? I dance every single day, even if it's just in my living room with the music turned up loud. Few things make me feel as happy or as free. How does dancing make you feel? Do you dance as often as you could?

LESSON LEARNED

Dance often and much. It feels good and frees your soul.

Easy Pasta Salad with Grape Tomatoes and Chickpeas

In Italy, a typical meal often consists of pasta tossed with fresh, raw ingredients such as tomatoes and basil. This recipe follows the same principle: You cook the pasta, but not the ingredients that go with it. It's a fresh-tasting dish that can be enjoyed as soon as it's ready, but it's also the perfect make-ahead lunch for work or school. Just refrigerate it in an airtight container and enjoy it all week long. It's a super-nutritious and delicious alternative to sandwiches made with cold cuts. Your whole family will love it! The moms on my street take it to work and send it to school with their kids all the time. This recipe is also one I developed while working on a campaign with Catelli Healthy Harvest® Whole-grain Pasta. Enjoy! **SERVES 6**

1. Cook the pasta in boiling water according to the package instructions.
2. Meanwhile, in a large bowl, combine the grape tomatoes, basil, red onion, and chickpeas.
3. When the pasta is cooked, drain and rinse under cold running water. Add the pasta to the tomato and chickpea mixture. Set aside.
4. In a small bowl, whisk together the dressing ingredients (or put them in a small jar with a tight-fitting lid and shake well).
5. Gently toss the salad with the dressing and serve immediately or refrigerate in an airtight container to enjoy as a cold pasta salad later.

TIPS

- For a more kid-friendly version, use 2 green onions (white and green parts) instead of the red onion. Green onions are milder in flavour.

PER SERVING (2 CUPS/500 ML) 376 calories • 12 g fat • 2 g saturated fat • 58 g carbohydrate • 9 g fibre • 8 g sugars • 11 g protein • 316 g sodium

SALAD

6 cups (1.5 L) whole-wheat pasta bows

2 cups (500 mL) grape tomatoes, halved

1 cup (250 mL) loosely packed fresh basil leaves, chopped

¾ cup (185 mL) red onion, chopped

1 can (19 oz/540 mL) chickpeas, drained and rinsed

DRESSING

¼ cup (60 mL) extra virgin olive oil

3 Tbsp (45 mL) balsamic vinegar

2 Tbsp (30 mL) freshly squeezed lemon juice

1 Tbsp (15 mL) pure maple syrup

2 cloves garlic, minced

1 Tbsp (15 mL) Dijon mustard

1 teaspoon (5 mL) Worcestershire sauce

½ tsp (2.5 mL) salt

¼ tsp (1 mL) freshly ground black pepper

WHY RELATIONSHIPS FAIL, INCLUDING MARRIAGES

> "A 'no' uttered from the deepest conviction is better than a 'yes' merely uttered to please, or worse, to avoid trouble." **MAHATMA GANDHI**

WHY DO ROMANTIC or love relationships, including marriages, fail? Here's one big reason: lack of honesty. People are not honest about who they are, what they want, or what they need. As a result, the relationship is built on a shaky foundation. Honesty is the backbone of living life well and this includes loving well. In the beginning of a relationship people often pretend to be someone they're not (in some cases it's because they don't know who they are, which is equally dangerous). They believe they have to be someone else, be someone better, or be someone different in order to be loved. They think that who they really are is simply not enough. Who we are is always enough, especially for the right person. Once in the relationship, people continue being dishonest. They mould themselves to suit someone else's wants and needs rather than staying true to what they really want and need. While this may work in the short term, it's disaster in the long term. Everyone deserves to have their wants and needs met—at least the ones that are really important to them. When the relationship starts to fail, which many do, no one wants to look at that either. By ignoring it they think it will simply go away. It won't. How honest are you in your significant relationships? Are your wants and needs being met? Are you staying true to who you are? Are you addressing what's not working?

LESSON LEARNED

Relationships, including marriage, fail because people fail to be honest about who they are and what they need. Be courageous. Build your relationships on a foundation of truth.

Mediterranean-Herbed Brown Rice and Lentil Salad

This colourful, hearty, and delicious salad comes from Amy Snider-Whitson who runs The Test Kitchen, a company that specializes in recipe development and a whole lot more. It can be served alone or as a side salad with grilled chicken or fish. It also keeps well in the refrigerator and makes a terrific, fibre-rich portable lunch option that will keep energy levels high all afternoon. I recommend using parboiled whole-grain brown rice (like Uncle Ben's) because it has a nice fluffy texture in salads, but you can use whatever brown rice you like. The lentils can be replaced with another canned legume such as chickpeas, navy beans, or black beans. You can add zest with a sprinkle of crumbled feta cheese before serving. This salad is fantastic. Thanks, Amy! Enjoy! **SERVES 4 TO 6**

1. In a large pot of boiling water, cook the rice according to the package instructions. Drain and spread out on a large plate to cool.
2. In a large bowl, toss the cooled rice with the lentils, red pepper, onion, and mixed herbs. Set aside.
3. In a small bowl, whisk together the vinegar, garlic, Dijon, oregano, honey, pepper, and salt. Whisking, drizzle in the oil until well combined.
4. Add the dressing to the rice mixture and toss to combine. Taste and adjust the seasonings, if needed. (If making ahead, hold back half of the dressing and add just before serving.).

TIP

- For extra protein and nutrition, you can add ¼ cup (60 mL) of toasted pine nuts or slivered almonds.

PER SERVING (1 CUP/250 ML) 276 calories · 14 g fat · 1 g saturated fat · 43 g carbohydrates · 3.5 g sugars · 5 g fibre · 9 g protein · 230 mg sodium

SALAD

1 cup (250 mL) whole-grain brown rice

1 can (19 oz/540 mg) lentils, drained and rinsed

1 cup (250 mL) diced red bell pepper

½ cup (125 mL) diced red onion

1½ cups (375 mL) chopped fresh mixed herbs (such as parsley, mint, and/or basil)

DRESSING

2 Tbsp (30 mL) red wine vinegar

1 large clove garlic, minced

1 Tbsp (15 mL) Dijon mustard

1 tsp (5 mL) dried oregano leaves

1 tsp (5 mL) liquid honey

¼ tsp (1 mL) freshly ground black pepper

Pinch of salt

3 Tbsp (45 mL) extra virgin olive oil

YOU ARE ENOUGH

"Live life. Be brave. Believe in yourself. Be kind to others. Smile daily. Love as much as possible, and always remember, you are enough." UNKNOWN

How would you feel if I told you that you are enough—completely, totally, and entirely enough? Let this sink into your soul. How does it make you feel? Does it provide relief of any kind? Is it even possible for you to fully believe? Unfortunately, everyone—to one degree or another—carries with them a belief that says "I am not enough. I have to do more, be more, and achieve more." This belief drains us of our energy and steals our joy. It's how we abuse and beat ourselves up every single day. It's like being on a treadmill we can't get off. Who wants that? Not me. What if you were to carry around a different belief, one that says "Right now, in this moment, today, I am enough, exactly as I am"? I've done enough. I've said enough. I've been enough. I'm right where I need to be. I don't need to do one thing more! This doesn't mean you give up on your dreams and goals. It doesn't mean you can't be more, do more, or achieve more in the future. What it does mean is that right now, in this moment, today, you are enough—completely, totally, and entirely enough—exactly as you are. This belief is one of the most beautiful and liberating beliefs I carry. I feel tremendous gratitude for it. What's more, when I really let it sink into my soul, that's when I also feel the most inspired and the most free to actually be all that I am capable of being.

LESSON LEARNED

When we accept ourselves as "enough," we free ourselves to be everything we are capable of being.

Indian-Spiced Brown Rice and Lentils

Lentils are a nutritional powerhouse loaded with folate, iron, potassium, and protein. A wonderful way to enjoy them is combined with brown rice. Add some kick-butt spices and you have one tasty and very nutritious meal. Enjoy either as a side dish or as the main meal. It also makes a great brown-bag lunch. **SERVES 2 TO 4**

1. In a medium pot over medium heat, heat the oil. Add the onion and sauté until just starting to turn golden brown, 3 to 4 minutes. Add the garlic and sauté for another 30 seconds.
2. Remove the pot from the heat and add the cumin, cinnamon, cloves, turmeric, and dried red peppers flakes. Mix well.
3. Return the pot to the heat, stirring continuously so the spices don't burn. Add the broth, lentils, and rice. Bring to a simmer. Cover and reduce the heat to low. Simmer until the lentils and rice are tender and the liquid is absorbed, 20 to 25 minutes.
4. Turn off the heat. Stir in the cilantro and lemon zest. Let sit for a few minutes. If desired, serve sprinkled with Parmesan.

TIPS

- I use parboiled brown rice (such as Uncle Ben's) in this recipe. It cooks in 20 to 25 minutes, which is the same amount of time it takes for the lentils to cook. If you use regular brown rice (which takes about 45 minutes to cook), add the lentils after the brown rice has already been cooking for about 20 minutes.
- If you're not a fan of turmeric (which gives the dish a curry-like flavour), omit it and double up on the cumin instead.
- For extra sweetness and goodness, add ¼ cup (60 mL) of raisins or currants.

PER SERVING (¾ CUP/185 mL) 215 calories · 4.6 g fat · 0.7 g saturated fat · 35 g carbohydrates · 1 g sugars · 9 g fibre · 8.5 g protein · 50 g sodium

1 Tbsp (15 mL) extra virgin olive oil

1 medium onion, diced

2 cloves, garlic, minced

1 tsp (5 mL) ground cumin

1 tsp (5 mL) ground cinnamon

1 tsp (5 mL) ground cloves

½ tsp (2.5 mL) turmeric

½ tsp (2.5 mL) dried red pepper flakes

2 cups (500 mL) lower-sodium chicken broth

½ cup (125 mL) dried green lentils, rinsed and drained

½ cup (125 mL) brown rice

½ cup (125 mL) chopped fresh cilantro leaves

1 tsp (5 mL) freshly grated lemon peel (zest)

Freshly grated Parmesan cheese (optional)

LET GO, SURRENDER, AND TASTE FREEDOM

> "When I let go of what I am, I become what I might be. When I let go of what I have, I receive what I need." **TAO TE CHING**

THINK ABOUT THE difference between hanging on and letting go. Which do you think is easier to do? Logic tells me it should be far easier to let go. To hang on to anything requires effort. Experience, however, has taught me that letting go sometimes feels impossible. Why? In most cases, it's because we fear what will happen if we do. Will our world fall apart? Will we be okay? Many of us hang on to things way longer than we should. We hang on to bad habits. We hang on to limiting beliefs. We hang on to unhealthy relationships. We even hang on to stuff around our house that we don't want or need. Hanging on steals our peace, our serenity, and a whole lot of our energy. In many ways it steals our life. When we let go, we become free. We are free to live life on our own terms and to make our lives what we want them to be. Make a list of all the things you're hanging on to that don't contribute positively to your life. Imagine letting each and every one of those things go. Don't you feel lighter already?

LESSON LEARNED

Get good at letting go, especially of those things that don't serve you well, such as unhealthy relationships, limiting beliefs, and bad habits. Free yourself to make your life all that you want it to be.

Tuscan Supper

My friend and the co-author of my last two books, Mairlyn Smith, recently released a new cookbook called Healthy Starts Here. *All the recipes in her book are super healthy and super delicious! Mairlyn, without question, is a master chef in the kitchen. She has many devoted fans for good reason. This dish is made with barley, which is good for gut health, healthy blood sugar, and lowering cholesterol. It's also very satisfying and keeps you feeling full for a long time. Serve it with grilled chicken or fish. Thanks, Mairlyn! Enjoy!* **SERVES 6**

1 Tbsp (15 mL) extra virgin olive oil

1 onion, diced

4 large cloves garlic, minced

4 cups (1 L) sliced cremini mushrooms (about 24 mushrooms)

1 Tbsp (15 mL) dried basil

1 tsp (5 mL) dried oregano leaves

¼ tsp (1 mL) freshly ground black pepper

1 cup (250 mL) pot barley, rinsed and drained

1 can (19 oz/540 mL) diced tomatoes

1 cup (250 mL) lower-sodium vegetable or chicken broth

½ cup (125 mL) grated Asiago, Parmesan, or pecorino cheese, divided

1. Heat a large pot over medium heat. Add the oil, then the onion, and sauté until golden brown, about 5 minutes. (This extra bit of time browning the onion pays off in the end as it gives the dish a deeper flavour.)

2. Add the garlic and mushrooms and sauté for 3 minutes.

3. Add the basil, oregano, and pepper, and sauté for 1 minute. Add the barley and sauté for 1 minute.

4. Stir in the tomatoes and broth, making sure you scrape up all the little browned bits stuck to the bottom of the pot.

5. Bring to a boil and stir again. Reduce the heat to a simmer and cook, covered, until the barley is cooked through and soft but not mushy, 45 to 50 minutes. Stir occasionally and adjust the heat so it doesn't burn.

6. Remove from the heat, stir once, and let sit, covered, for 10 minutes. Spoon into bowls and top each serving with 2 Tbsp (30 mL) grated cheese.

TIP

• If you want to use fresh herbs instead of dried, substitute 3 Tbsp (45 mL) of chopped fresh basil and 1 Tbsp (15 mL) of chopped fresh oregano, but add them just before serving so the flavour isn't completely cooked out of the herbs.

PER SERVING (1 CUP/250 ML) 207 calories • 5 g total fat • 1 g saturated fat • 33 g carbohydrates • 5.5 g sugars • 8 g fibre • 9 g protein • 309 mg sodium

LET ME HOLD YOU AND CARRY YOU GENTLY

> "Our prime purpose in this life is to help others. And if you can't help them, at least don't hurt them."
>
> **DALAI LAMA**

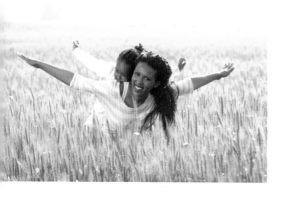

IHAVE A VERY special place in my heart for children who grow up in homes that are lacking in love, caring, attention, and affection. These are things all children need to thrive and to be their best. These children grow up feeling alone, scared, and broken, sometimes into a million tiny pieces. Some of these children are fortunate to get the help they need to heal. Others are not so lucky. Did you grow up in such a home? Do you know someone who did? If you know such a person, I ask you to hold and carry these wounded souls gently in your heart. Let them know you love them. Communicate true compassion for their pain and suffering. Let them know they've done enough. They suffered enough, struggled enough, and hurt enough. They are enough, just as they are. You don't need them to be or do anything more. This is what these wounded souls need and deserve. They deserve to be held and gently carried in our hearts today and always.

LESSON LEARNED

Broken childhoods often result in broken children who grow up to be broken adults. Hold and carry these wounded souls gently in your heart. They deserve our love, compassion, and kindness always.

Mushroom Quinoa Risotto

My friend and the co-author of my last two books, Mairlyn Smith, got together with a group of professional home economists to write The Vegetarian's Complete Quinoa Cookbook. *It's a wonderful book of healthy, tasty recipes. Rosemarie Superville developed this creamy and delicious risotto. Guess what it's made of? Quinoa! For extra-special flavour, use a mixture of wild mushrooms. Thanks, Rosemarie, Mairlyn, and the rest of the team! Enjoy!* **SERVES 4**

1. Place the quinoa in a large saucepan. Add 2 cups (500 mL) of the broth and bring to a boil over medium-high heat. Reduce the heat to medium-low and cook, covered, until the quinoa grains are translucent and most of the liquid has been absorbed, 10 to 15 minutes.
2. Meanwhile, in a large non-stick frying pan, heat the oil over medium heat. Add the onion and sauté until softened, about 2 minutes.
3. Add the mushrooms and cook, stirring occasionally, until browned and juicy, about 5 minutes.
4. Add the garlic, thyme, and flour. Cook, stirring, for another minute.
5. Stir in the cooked quinoa, vinegar, and enough of the reserved broth to make the mixture creamy. (If you want it really creamy, add all of the remaining ¼ cup/60 mL of broth.)
6. Remove from heat. Stir in the Parmesan. Season with pepper. Serve immediately.

TIP
- To cut down on sodium, choose a sodium-reduced vegetable broth.

PER SERVING (1 CUP/250 ML) 274 calories • 8 g fat • 2 g saturated fat • 41 g carbohydrates • 5 g sugars • 5 g fibre • 11 g protein • 369 mg sodium

1 cup (250 mL) quinoa, rinsed and drained

2¼ cups (560 mL) vegetable broth, divided

1 Tbsp (15 mL) extra virgin olive oil

1 onion, diced

8 oz (230 g) cremini mushrooms, thinly sliced (about 3 cups/750 mL)

3 cloves garlic, minced

2 tsp (10 mL) chopped fresh thyme leaves

1 Tbsp (15 mL) whole-wheat flour

1 Tbsp (15 mL) balsamic vinegar

¼ cup (60 mL) freshly grated Parmesan cheese

Freshly ground black pepper, to taste

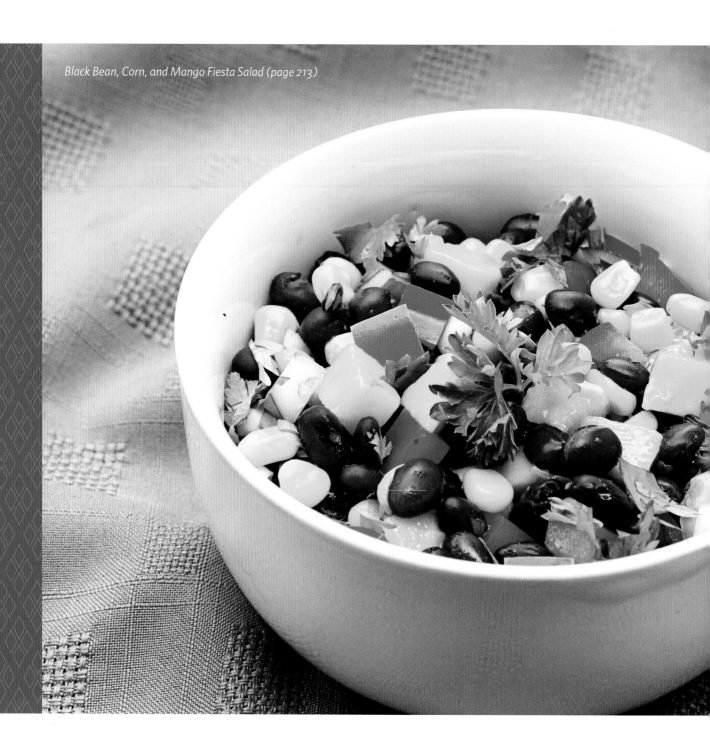

Black Bean, Corn, and Mango Fiesta Salad (page 213)

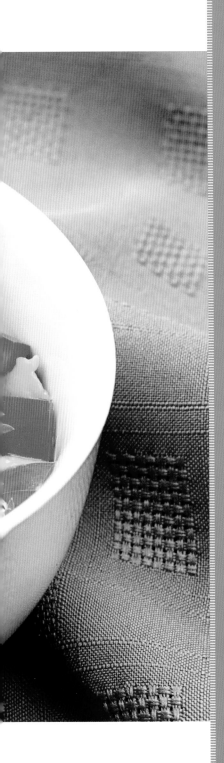

BEANS AND OTHER LEGUMES

*A life lesson comes with
every recipe. Enjoy!*

LIVING THE GOOD LIFE

> "It's not living that matters, but living rightly." **SOCRATES**

IN JANUARY 2011, my brother's youngest son, Aaron, started out on the trip of a lifetime. At the age of 25, single and having just finished training to be a chef, he decided to take a year to travel throughout New Zealand before settling down. He spent the first four months with no set itinerary, stopping in different places and staying for as long as it felt good to stay. Then he came to Raglan, a small, beautiful, beachside town known for its surfing. This is where he lived for the next eight months. He got a job at the local hostel. He spent each morning working at reception checking in new guests and showing them around (the maximum length of stay was two weeks, so lots of people passed through). Everyone he met and worked with was incredibly interesting, so happy, and had a positive outlook on life. The scenery was beyond breathtaking. The best part of the day, however, was the afternoon. Aaron spent each afternoon riding the waves and learning how to surf like nobody's business. "There's no feeling like it. You're part of the elements, part of the ocean. It's so physical. It's pure exhilaration!" was how Aaron described it. When I saw the video of Aaron surfing (he had a special camera that had been sent to him by his sister mounted on his board), it made me cry. He looked so happy and alive. This was really living! Isn't that what life is for?

LESSON LEARNED

Life is meant for living. It's meant for new and different and exciting. It's meant for happy and beautiful and exhilarating. It's meant for people and love and laughter. Make your life all this and more!

P.S. In February 2013, Aaron left to spend another year in Raglan where, once again, he was happy, free, and totally alive. Aaron knows what it means to live the good life.

Black Bean, Corn, and Mango Fiesta Salad

This colourful, fresh salad is so delicious you'll find it hard to stop eating it once you start. It's one of those dishes that if you bring it to a party, someone will definitely ask you for the recipe. Loaded with super-nutritious, antioxidant-rich, disease-fighting ingredients—black beans, mango, and red pepper—your body will jump up and down with joy when you eat it and so will your taste buds. Enjoy! **SERVES 6**

1. In a large bowl, combine the salad ingredients. Set aside.
2. In a small bowl, whisk together the dressing ingredients, only adding the salt if you are using unsalted beans and corn.
3. Pour the dressing over the salad and stir until combined.

TIPS

- I recommend using Ataulfo mangoes (they have the fully yellow skin). You'll need 2 for this recipe.
- If you'd like to give the salad some extra kick, add some of the seeds from the jalapeño pepper. The more seeds you add, the hotter it will be!
- This recipe is super versatile: Serve it as a side salad with grilled chicken or fish, as an appetizer with baked tortilla chips, or as a main course as a wrap (wrap with romaine lettuce leaves or whole-grain tortillas).

PER SERVING (1 CUP/250 ML) 162 calories · 3.5 g fat · 0.5 g saturated fat · 29 g carbohydrates · 11 g sugars · 6 g fibre · 6 g protein · 110 mg sodium

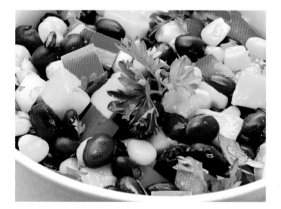

SALAD

1 can (19 oz/540 mL) black beans (no salt added), drained and rinsed

1 can (12 oz/355 mL) corn (no salt added), drained

1½ cups (375 mL) diced mango

1 small red bell pepper, diced

1 small red onion, finely diced

1 jalapeño pepper (seeds removed), finely diced

⅓ cup (80 mL) chopped fresh cilantro leaves

⅓ cup (80 mL) chopped fresh parsley leaves

DRESSING

1 Tbsp (15 mL) extra virgin olive oil

1 Tbsp (15 mL) freshly squeezed lime juice

1 Tbsp (15 mL) balsamic vinegar

1 clove garlic, minced

1 tsp (5 mL) chili powder

½ tsp (2.5 mL) ground cumin

¼ tsp (1 mL) salt (optional)

SING YOUR HEART OUT

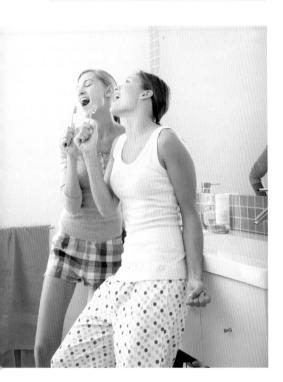

> "If I cannot fly, let me sing."
>
> **STEPHEN SONDHEIM**

THE OTHER DAY I was on an airplane. A mother and her little girl sat down in the seats behind me. For almost the entire flight the girl sang. She sang song after song after song. She was a happy, sweet, singing girl. It's hard not to be happy when you're singing! I believe we were born to sing, whether we have a good voice or not. It's such a joyful thing to do. That's why I sing often (and I'm not a good singer!). I sing in my house. I sing in my car. I sing when I'm dancing (and usually lose my voice in the process). Singing makes me feel free and definitely alive—especially when I really belt it out. How often do you sing? Do you really let yourself go? Wouldn't you love to be the lead singer in a band or perhaps a back-up singer (at least in your dreams)? I encourage you to leave lots of room in your life for singing. Sing regularly. Sing often. Sing loudly. Just sing!

LESSON LEARNED

Few things in life feel as wonderful as singing. Let yourself feel wonderful today. Sing and sing and sing and sing!

P.S. Ella Fitzgerald said, "The only thing better than singing, is more singing!"

Warm Lentil Salad with Feta and Fresh Herbs

Lentils are a nutritional goldmine, chock full of protein, B vitamins, and fibre. In this recipe I combine them with super-nutritious carrots, red peppers, and spinach. What really makes this dish wonderful, however, is adding the feta cheese to the warm salad at the end. The first time my girlfriend Teri tested this recipe for me, she simply couldn't stop eating it. I hope you love it as much as she did. Enjoy! **SERVES 2 TO 4**

1. In a large frying pan or skillet over medium heat, heat the oil. Add the onion and sauté until softened, about 3 minutes.
2. Add the carrots and red pepper and sauté just until tender-crisp, 2 to 3 minutes. Add the garlic and sauté for another 30 seconds.
3. Add the lentils and spinach and sauté until the lentils are just heated through and the spinach is wilted, 1 to 2 minutes. Stir in the basil, parsley, vinegar, and pepper. Transfer to a large bowl.
4. Add the feta. Stir gently to combine. Serve immediately.

TIPS
- You can substitute an equal amount of light goat cheese for the feta cheese.
- For extra kick, add ¼ tsp (1 mL) dried red pepper flakes.

PER SERVING (¾ CUP/185 ML) 207 calories • 9.5 g fat • 2.5 g saturated fat • 22 g carbohydrates • 5 g sugars • 10 g fibre • 10 g protein • 294 mg sodium

2 Tbsp (30 mL) extra virgin olive oil

1 onion, diced

2 medium carrots, finely diced

1 small red bell pepper, finely diced

1 clove garlic, minced

1 can (19 oz/540 mL) lentils, drained and rinsed

3 cups (750 mL) loosely packed baby spinach

¼ cup (60 mL) chopped fresh basil leaves

¼ cup (60 mL) chopped fresh parsley leaves

2 Tbsp (30 mL) balsamic vinegar

¼ tsp (1 mL) freshly ground black pepper

⅓ cup (80 mL) crumbled light feta cheese

LOVE IS NOT LOGICAL

LOVE IS MANY things: wonderful, exhilarating, terrifying, uplifting, joyful, an inspiration. Love, however, is definitely not logical. Matters of the heart never are. Your heart feels what it wants to feel and it feels it deeply. Your brain can try to override your heart, but when it comes to love, good luck. When you love somebody, you love somebody. Even if you shouldn't love them or wish you didn't love them—and even if they don't love you. You can't stop love, especially intense love. It's like a train on a track going full speed. You might be able to slow it down, but usually that's about the best you can do. Love can be crazy, foolish, and totally impractical. What's the lesson here? Accept it. Understand it. Know it. This doesn't mean you run off with the mailman because you've fallen in love with him (although it may be what you need to do). It just means you don't deny the love you feel. You don't pretend it isn't there. That doesn't help anyone. See it, feel it, taste it. Then figure out what you are—or are not—going to do about it. Just remember, don't expect love to play nice, be fair, or do exactly what you want it to do. Love just doesn't work that way. Love is beautiful, but logical it's not!

LESSON LEARNED

Don't expect love to be rational, sane, or logical in any way. See it and feel it for what it is. What you do about what you feel . . . well, that's up to you!

Liz's Award-Winning Chili

If you're wondering who decided this chili recipe was worthy of an award ... it was me! I gave it an award because it's that delicious. I love it, my kids love it, and my neighbours and their kids love it. I think you will, too! Bonus: It's loaded with disease-fighting, fibre-rich beans. Make it on the weekend so you can let it simmer on low heat for at least 3 to 4 hours. It tastes best this way. If you prefer a vegetarian version, omit the ground beef and add an extra can of beans. The meat, however, provides an excellent source of easily absorbed iron and zinc—two nutrients that most women in particular don't get enough of. Enjoy! **SERVES 8**

1. In a large frying pan over medium heat, cook the ground beef for 5 to 8 minutes or until no longer pink, breaking it into small pieces while cooking. Drain off all of the fat (discard the fat) and set the meat aside.

2. In a large pot over medium heat, heat the oil. Add the onions and sauté until soft and translucent, 3 to 5 minutes. Add the garlic and sauté for another 30 seconds.

3. Add the cooked meat, tomatoes, black beans, kidney beans, maple syrup, chili powder, Worcestershire sauce, cumin, oregano, pepper and red pepper flakes. Only add salt if you used canned tomatoes that contain no added salt.

4. Bring to a boil. Reduce the heat to low and simmer, uncovered, for at least 3 to 4 hours, until nicely thickened. (Stir regularly while cooking.) To serve, ladle into bowls and top with cheese (if using).

TIP

- If you prefer a smoky-flavoured chili, reduce the amount of chili powder to 1 Tbsp (15 mL) and add 1 Tbsp (15 mL) chipotle chili powder.

PER SERVING (1½ CUPS/375 ML) 314 calories • 8.5 g fat •
2.5 g saturated fat • 42 g carbohydrates • 8 g sugars • 8 g fibre •
25 g protein • 395 mg sodium

1 lb (500 g) extra lean ground beef

2 Tbsp (30 mL) extra virgin olive oil

2 medium onions, chopped

4 cloves garlic, minced

2 cans (28 oz/796 mL) diced tomatoes (no salt added)

1 can (19 oz/540 mL) black beans (no salt added), drained and rinsed

1 can (19 oz/540 mL) kidney beans (no salt added), drained and rinsed

1 Tbsp (15 mL) pure maple syrup

2 Tbsp (30 mL) chili powder

1 Tbsp (15 mL) Worcestershire sauce

1 tsp (5 mL) ground cumin

1 tsp (5 mL) dried oregano leaves

½ tsp (2.5 mL) freshly ground black pepper

¼ tsp (1 mL) dried red pepper flakes

1 tsp (5 mL) salt

Freshly grated Parmesan or aged cheddar cheese (optional)

SAYING GOODBYE WITH LOVE

> "There is a sacredness in tears. They are not the mark of weakness, but of power. They speak more eloquently than ten thousand tongues. They are messengers of overwhelming grief . . . and of unspeakable love."
>
> **WASHINGTON IRVING**

I RECEIVED A TEXT from my oldest daughter, Chelsea, while she was away at university. She had just received news that a man she had worked very closely with at camp over several summers had died. His name was Trevor. He was 55 years old and married with children and grandchildren. He'd fallen from a ladder. My daughter was very upset. She described Trevor as the nicest man she'd ever met in her entire life. This is the advice I gave my daughter: Feel your loss and feel it completely. That's how you honour the people you lose. Cry. Scream. Write about it. Talk about it. Do whatever feels good and right to you. Immerse yourself in who he was and all that he represented. Don't deny any of it. Not one single drop. Stand fully in the love you feel. Celebrate him and all that he gave. Do this for as long as it takes and as long as you need to. There are no rules, no rights or wrongs, when it comes to loss, love, and grieving. Accept his death. Why he had to go you may never fully comprehend, but he did and you can't change that he is gone. Feeling our loss is how I believe we best honour those who die.

LESSON LEARNED

The best way to honour those who die is to stand fully in how you feel about their death. To acknowledge all that they were, all that they are, and all that they ever will be to you.

Amazing Black Bean Quesadillas

If you don't have my last book, Ultimate Foods for Ultimate Health, *I strongly suggest you pick one up (it's a national bestselling award-winner). It contains lots of great nutrition information, and my co-author, Mairlyn Smith, did an exceptional job on all of the recipes. This is one of my favourites. It's a delicious way to get more fibre and antioxidant-rich black beans into your eating plan—and your whole family will enjoy it.* **SERVES 5**

2 tsp (10 mL) extra virgin olive oil

1 onion, diced

1 red bell pepper, diced

2 cloves garlic, minced

½ tsp (2.5 mL) ground cumin

1 can (19 oz/540 mL) black beans (no salt added), drained and rinsed

1 cup (250 mL) salsa (mild, medium, or hot)

5 large whole-wheat soft flour tortillas

½ cup (125 mL) shredded light Monterey Jack cheese

1. In a large frying pan over medium heat, heat the oil. Add the onion and red pepper and sauté until the veggies are soft, about 3 minutes. Add the garlic and sauté for another 30 seconds.

2. Add the cumin, beans, and salsa. Stir well. When the beans are heated through, remove from the heat. (This can be made ahead of time and stored in an airtight container in the refrigerator for up to 3 days.)

3. Preheat the oven to 350°F (175°C). Put a baking sheet in the oven.

4. Heat a frying pan over medium heat. Place 1 tortilla in the pan. Spoon ¾ cup (185 mL) of the bean mixture on one half. Sprinkle with 2 Tbsp (30 mL) of the cheese. Fold the other half of the tortilla over the beans and press down gently with a spatula. Brown the underside (this takes about 1 minute) and then very carefully flip it over to brown the other side.

5. When the tortilla is cooked, transfer it to the baking sheet in the oven. Repeat with the remaining quesadillas.

6. To serve, cut each tortilla into 4 triangles. Serve with salsa and low-fat sour cream, if desired.

TIP

• The sodium content of salsa and tortillas varies considerably from one brand to the next. Make lower-sodium choices.

PER QUESADILLA 280 calories • 6 g fat • 2.5 g saturated fat • 45 g carbohydrates • 4 g sugars • 9 g fibre • 14 g protein • 475 mg sodium

KISSING MAKES LIFE MORE DELICIOUS!

"I believe in pink. I believe that laughing is the best calorie burner. I believe in kissing, kissing a lot. I believe in being strong when everything seems to be going wrong. I believe that happy girls are the prettiest girls. I believe that tomorrow is another day and I believe in miracles."

AUDREY HEPBURN

IF YOU ARE married, have a special someone in your life, or soon hope to have a special someone in your life, then this is for you. It's about kissing. When was the last time you shared a really wonderful, knock-'em-dead, all-out kiss with your partner? I'm not talking about a peck on the cheek. I'm talking about a real kiss—a passionate, beautiful, amazing, incredible kiss! I think kissing makes life way more delicious and most of us don't do enough of it. We do a lot of kissing at the beginning of our relationships, but as time goes by, kissing just isn't the priority it used to be. One of my most memorable days was spent by a riverbank kissing my childhood sweetheart for a whole afternoon. What a beautiful afternoon that was! So here's the question: If you knew you had just one day left to live, wouldn't you want at least one more awesomely wonderful kiss in your life? I would. What's stopping you from enjoying one today? Or even every day?

LESSON LEARNED

Great kissing makes life more wonderful. Kiss (I mean really kiss!) your spouse, partner, or lover today (and every day!).

Rosemary Roasted Chickpeas

If you're looking for an awesomely delicious and totally nutritious snack or mini meal, look no further. One of the tastiest ways to enjoy chickpeas is to roast them. Chickpeas, like all beans, are nutritional all-stars, disease-fighting superstars, and fibre mega-stars. I make this recipe at least once a week. My daughter and I often have this for dinner along with some raw veggies and dip or a salad. I wouldn't be surprised if after you try them, they become a weekly part of your eating plan as well. They're that good. Enjoy! **MAKES ABOUT 2 CUPS (500 ML)**

1 can (19 oz/540 mL) chick-peas (no salt added), drained and rinsed

1 Tbsp (15 mL) extra virgin olive oil

2 tsp (10 mL) dried rosemary

½ tsp (2.5 mL) salt

¼ tsp (1 mL) freshly ground black pepper

1. Preheat the oven to 350° F (175°C).
2. In a medium bowl, combine all of the ingredients.
3. Spread the chickpea mixture in an even layer on a baking sheet lined with parchment paper and bake for 40 to 45 minutes. The chickpeas should be golden brown, slightly crunchy on the outside, and slightly soft on the inside. If they are hard crunchy, you have overcooked them.
4. Enjoy them hot just out of the oven. They taste best this way!

TIP

- If you are using chickpeas that already have salt added, either omit the salt in this recipe entirely or only add about ¼ tsp (1 mL).

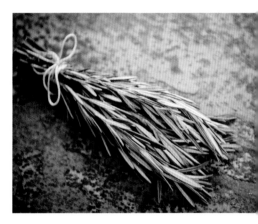

PER SERVING (½ CUP/125 ML) 200 calories • 5.5 g fat • 0.5 g saturated fat • 29 g carbohydrates • 1 g sugars • 8 g fibre • 10 g protein • 293 mg sodium

MEDITATION CAN TRANSFORM YOUR LIFE, IF YOU LET IT

> "Generally we waste our lives, distracted from our true selves, in endless activity. Meditation is the way to bring us back to ourselves, where we can really experience and taste our full being."
>
> **SOGYAL RINPOCHE**

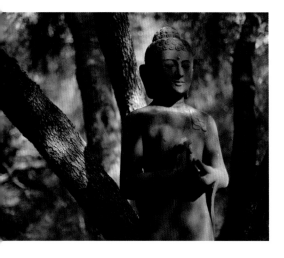

ALMOST TWO YEARS ago I got serious about meditation. I made a decision to make it a regular part of my life. To say that it has changed my life is an understatement—it has transformed it. I believe it can do the same for you, if you let it.

What do you gain by sitting with yourself in silence every day?

- You get to truly know yourself. You get to hear, see, feel, and connect with who you are and what you need on a much deeper level.
- You learn the art of letting go. This is huge. In a true meditation, as thoughts enter your mind, you observe them, but don't hang on to them. This builds up your "letting go" muscle and serves you well in daily life. It helps you to let go of anger, hurt, sadness, and resentments—even those you've carried for a lifetime. Chaos can surround you, but you can choose not to be part of it. Nothing has to disturb your peace of mind, if you don't want it to.
- You connect to your own heart. Your heart is honest and speaks only truth. It leads you to happiness and joy. It teaches you about love. You come to know that love truly is all that matters.

I encourage you make room in your life for meditation. Give it the respect it deserves. Commit to it. Allow it to change your life. It will, if you let it.

LESSON LEARNED

Meditation can transform your life. It teaches you about who you are, what you need, letting go, peace, serenity, connection, safety, and love. It teaches you how to live—there is no more valuable lesson.

Honey-Roasted Spiced Lentils

Lentils are a goldmine of nutrition. They're absolutely loaded with fibre and rich in protein, B vitamins (especially folate), iron, copper, and potassium. A great way to enjoy them is roasted. They make a far healthier snack than potato chips or pretzels. Kids like them, too—at least the kids on my street do! **SERVES 4**

1 Tbsp (15 mL) extra virgin olive oil

1 tsp (5 mL) liquid honey

1 tsp (5 mL) chili powder

½ tsp (2.5 mL) dried oregano

½ tsp (2.5 mL) ground cumin

1 can (19 oz/540 mL) lentils, drained and rinsed

1. Preheat the oven to 425°F (220°C).
2. In a medium bowl, whisk together the oil, honey, chili powder, oregano, and cumin. Add the lentils and mix to combine.
3. Spread the lentil mixture in an even layer on a baking sheet lined with parchment paper and bake for 20 to 25 minutes or until lightly crisped.
4. Enjoy hot just out of the oven. They taste best this way!

TIP
- This spice mixture works well on roasted chickpeas, too!

PER SERVING (½ CUP/125 ML) 159 calories • 4 g fat • 0.5 g saturated fat • 23 g carbohydrates • 2.5 g sugars • 5 g fibre • 8 g protein • 100 mg sodium

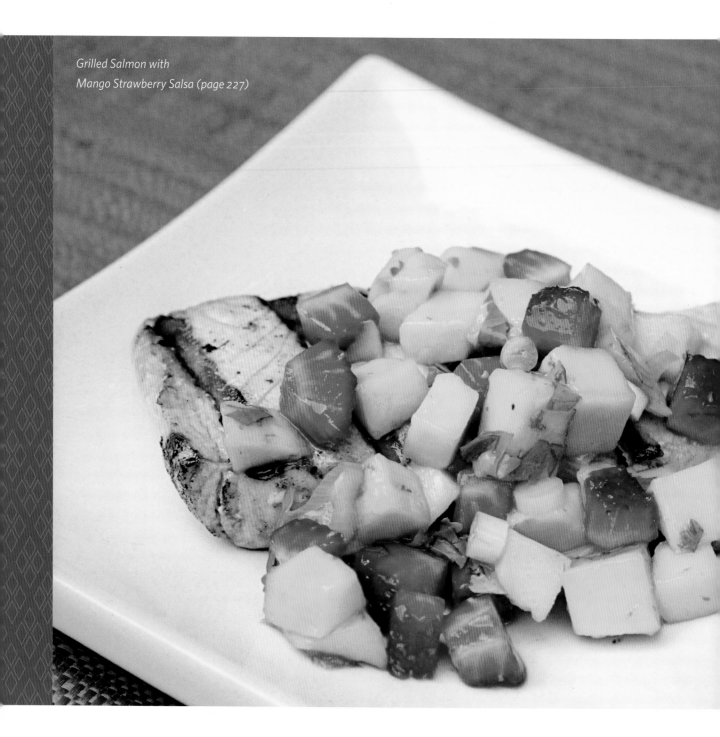

Grilled Salmon with
Mango Strawberry Salsa (page 227)

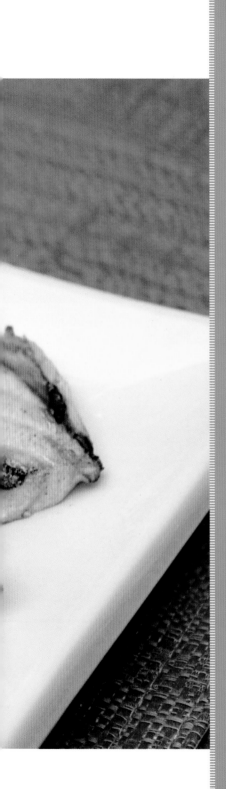

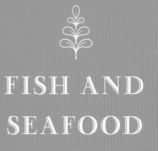

FISH AND SEAFOOD

*A life lesson comes with
every recipe. Enjoy!*

A LOVE LETTER FROM THE HEART

> "You'll never regret writing any letter out of love." **MARY MATALIN**

THIS PAST YEAR I received news about a friend from high school I knew well. At the age of 52, he died suddenly of a heart attack. His family and friends were in shock. Although he was overweight and could have taken better care of himself, his death came unexpectedly. Many of those close to him have regrets. There are things they wanted to say to him—there are things they wanted to do with him—but now he's gone. What can we learn from this (other than taking care of our own health)? How can we make our own lives better, because of it? This is my challenge to you: Imagine for a moment that you have only one week left to live. Knowing this, you've made the decision to write letters to all the people in your life that you love the most. Each letter is a love letter from the heart, a letter that speaks intimately about what you feel—what you love most about each person and what they mean to you. What would you say? What would you most want each person to know? Here's the next challenge: Even though you're not going to die in a week (at least I hope not!), I want you to write these letters anyway. If your schedule is busy, consider writing one heartfelt letter each week or take a vacation just to write letters. Write letters to your spouse or partner, your parents, your kids, your siblings, and your closest friends. Take your time. Say the words that live in your heart. Hold nothing back. The rewards for doing so are beyond comprehension—for you and for them. You don't have to regret the words you didn't say. They get to hear the words that mean so much to hear.

LESSON LEARNED

Life is unpredictable. Never miss an opportunity to tell the people you love just how much you love them. Nothing is more important, more precious, or more life-giving than that.

Grilled Salmon with Mango Strawberry Salsa

The co-author of my last book, Mairlyn Smith, introduced me to mango salsa. Since then I have become a huge fan and have experimented with many versions. It's truly one of my favourite meal accompaniments. I love it served over grilled fish, especially salmon, but it's great with grilled chicken, too. This mango-strawberry combo is especially wonderful. I'm not sure there is a more delicious way to enjoy salmon. Try it today and serve it to company the next time they visit. Enjoy! **SERVES 4**

1. In a medium bowl, whisk together the lime zest and juice, oil, and garlic. Add the salmon, turning once to coat. Cover and refrigerate until ready to grill.
2. Meanwhile, in a small bowl, combine all of the salsa ingredients. Let sit at room temperature, covered, until serving time.
3. Preheat the grill to medium heat. Spray with non-stick vegetable oil. Place the salmon on the grill and season lightly with salt (if using) and pepper. Close the lid and cook for 3 to 5 minutes per side (depending on the thickness of each fillet) or until the fish flakes easily with a fork (only turn the fish once).
4. Transfer the salmon to four serving plates and top with equal amounts of the salsa. Serve with brown rice or quinoa.

TIPS

- For best results, marinate the salmon and prepare the salsa 30 minutes to 8 hours prior to mealtime. Cover and refrigerate until ready to use.
- To kick things up a notch, add 1 finely diced jalapeño pepper, including the seeds. The more seeds you add, the hotter it will be!
- If you don't want to grill the salmon, simply bake it in the oven at 425°F (220°C) for 10 to 15 minutes or until it flakes easily with a fork.

PER SERVING (1 FILLET WITH ½ CUP/125 ML SALSA) 233 calories ·
10 g fat · 2 g saturated fat · 14 g carbohydrates · 10 g sugars ·
2 g fibre · 22 g protein · 208 mg sodium

FISH

Grated peel (zest) and juice of 1 lime

1 tsp (5 mL) extra virgin olive oil

1 clove garlic, minced

4 salmon fillets (each about 3½ oz/100 g)

¼ tsp (1 mL) freshly ground black pepper

¼ tsp (1 mL) salt (optional)

SALSA

1½ cups (375 mL) diced mango

¾ cup (185 mL) diced strawberries

1 green onion, chopped (white and green parts)

3 Tbsp (45 mL) chopped fresh cilantro leaves

Grated peel (zest) and juice of 1 lime

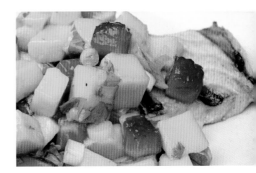

DON'T PRETEND TO BE HAPPY IF YOU'RE NOT

> "We are so accustomed to disguise ourselves to others that in the end we become disguised to ourselves."
>
> **FRANÇOIS DE LA ROCHEFOUCAULD**

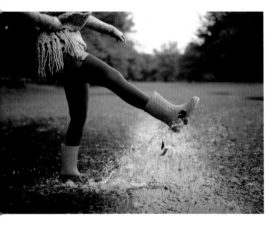

IT TAKES A tremendous amount of energy to pretend. It takes almost no energy to be who you are and to feel what you really feel. Young kids play pretend games, but they don't pretend about what they're thinking and what they're feeling. They cry when they feel like crying and laugh when they feel like laughing. Many of us, once we reach adulthood, have learned to pretend to some degree or another. Some of us have got it down to a fine art. We pretend we're okay when we're not. We pretend we feel one thing when what we really feel is something entirely different. We pretend to agree with someone or something when we don't agree at all. Pretending is a form of denial. It's a way of not looking, of lying to ourselves and the people around us. When we pretend about our situation or our problems, we get pretend solutions or no solutions at all. When as parents we pretend, we teach our kids to pretend as well. Life is supposed to be real. It's supposed to have ups and downs and in-betweens. The more real and honest you are with life, the more real and honest your life will be. Have the courage to be real.

LESSON LEARNED

Don't pretend about who you are, what you think, or what you feel. Pretending steals your energy and your life. It steals you.

Quinoa and Garlic Ginger Shrimp Bowls

Fresh-tasting, totally delicious, fast, and easy! This meal is great for lunch or dinner, and company will love it, too. Shrimp is a lean source of protein and rich in nutrients, including selenium, vitamin B12, choline, magnesium, zinc, and copper. Although shrimp does contain cholesterol, for most people, in moderation, it can easily fit into a healthy diet. As for quinoa, it is considered a whole grain and is rich in disease-fighting antioxidants, magnesium, and folate. Enjoy! **SERVES 4**

1. In a pot of boiling water, cook the quinoa according to the package instructions.
2. Meanwhile, in a small bowl, whisk together the dressing ingredients. Set aside.
3. In a large frying pan over medium heat, heat the oil. Add the shrimp and ginger and stir-fry until the shrimp turns pink and is cooked through, 3 to 4 minutes. Add 1 tablespoon (15 mL) of the dressing along with the garlic and sauté for another 30 seconds. Remove from the heat.
4. To serve, divide the cooked quinoa evenly among four bowls (about ¾ cup/185 mL per bowl). Drizzle each bowl with 1 tablespoon (15 mL) of the remaining dressing and stir until combined. Top each bowl with equal amounts of the shrimp mixture, tomato, avocado, and cilantro.

TIPS

- To remove the residue that sometimes gives quinoa a slightly bitter taste, rinse it under cold running water before cooking. Gently rub the seeds together between your hands.
- You can easily substitute brown rice for quinoa if you prefer. Quinoa, however, has more nutrition.
- I use sweet cocktail tomatoes because I find they have great flavour all year round.

PER SERVING (2 CUPS/500 ML) 342 calories · 12 g fat · 2 g saturated fat · 41 g carbohydrates · 8 g sugars · 7 g fibre · 21 g protein · 415 mg sodium

SHRIMP BOWL

1 cup (250 mL) quinoa, rinsed and drained (makes about 3 cups/750 mL cooked)

1 Tbsp (15 mL) extra virgin olive oil

⅔ lb (350 g) medium shrimp, peeled and deveined, tails removed (thawed and rinsed if frozen)

1 Tbsp (15 mL) minced gingerroot

2 cloves garlic, minced

1 cup (250 mL) diced sweet cocktail tomatoes

1 small avocado, diced

½ cup (125 mL) chopped fresh cilantro leaves

DRESSING

4 tsp (20 mL) sodium-reduced soy sauce

4 tsp (20 mL) liquid honey

4 tsp (20 mL) rice vinegar

CHOOSE TO BE MAGNIFICENTLY FREE

> "The secret of happiness is freedom. The secret of freedom is courage."
>
> **THUCYDIDES**

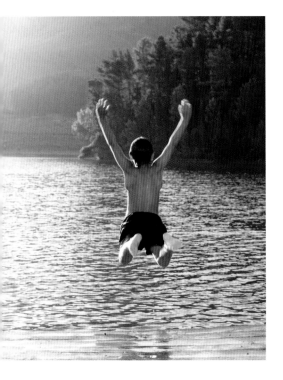

IF I TOLD you that you could be free—absolutely, totally, unequivocally, magnificently, and amazingly free—how would you feel? Would you feel liberated? Lighter? Would you feel happier and more joyful? Imagine if I told you that you could do whatever you wanted to do, go wherever you wanted to go, love whomever you want to love, and just be whoever you wanted to be. No restrictions. No holding back. Just living and enjoying every single moment of every single day. Now here's the critical question: What's stopping you from being free? What walls or chains, restrictions or constraints, do you put upon yourself? How do you hold yourself back? I believe we all have much greater freedom than we recognize or take advantage of. Each of us has far more incredible choices in a day that we could make, but we don't. Even with obligations and responsibilities like mortgages and kids and husbands and wives, we can live our lives more freely than most of us do. I challenge you to be free today, to live your life on your own terms.

LESSON LEARNED

Freedom is a choice. Many of us don't recognize what an incredible choice it is and just how much freedom we really have. Choose to be free today.

Grilled Salmon with Maple, Cumin, and Lime Marinade

Promise me that the next time you decide to throw some salmon on the grill you'll try this recipe. I think you'll thank me for it! Salmon is a disease-fighting powerhouse. It's good for your heart, brain, and eyes, and should make an appearance on your plate at least twice a week. This is an awesome recipe that everyone in your family will love—at least everyone in my family does. Enjoy! **SERVES 4**

1. In a medium bowl, whisk together all of the marinade ingredients.
2. Add the salmon to the marinade and turn to coat. Cover and refrigerate for about 30 minutes (you can also marinate the fish in a resealable bag).
3. Preheat the grill to medium heat. Spray with non-stick vegetable oil. Place the fillets on the grill and close the lid. Cook for 3 to 5 minutes per side (depending on the thickness of each fillet) or until the fish flakes easily with a fork. (Only turn the fish once.)
4. Serve with grilled veggies or a salad and brown rice or quinoa.

TIPS

- You can substitute an equal amount of fresh lemon juice for the lime juice.
- For extra flavour, try adding 1 tablespoon (15 mL) of chopped fresh cilantro leaves to the marinade.
- If you don't want to grill the salmon, simply bake it in the oven at 425°F (220°C) for 10 to 15 minutes or until it flakes easily with a fork.

PER SERVING (1 FILLET) 194 calories · 9 g fat · 2 g saturated fat · 6 g carbohydrates · 3 g sugars · 1 g fibre · 21 g protein · 270 mg sodium

MARINADE

Grated peel (zest) and juice of 1 lime

1 Tbsp (15 mL) Dijon mustard

1 Tbsp (15 mL) sodium-reduced soy sauce

1 Tbsp (15 mL) pure maple syrup

½ tsp (2.5 mL) ground cumin

¼ tsp (1 mL) freshly ground black pepper

1 clove garlic, minced

FISH

4 salmon fillets (each about 3½ oz/100 g)

A BELIEF THAT SETS YOU FREE

> "To err is human; to forgive, divine."
> **ALEXANDER POPE**

FORGIVENESS IS THE juice of life. When you forgive you don't have to carry around anger, bitterness, resentments, hate, sadness, or pain. Forgiveness, however, isn't always easy. We want people to pay for the hurt or harm we believe they cause. We hang on to the injustice of it all, sometimes as if our life depended on it. With forgiveness, however, we are rewarded with freedom, happiness, and joy—the things we really want. I have a simple but powerful belief that makes forgiveness easier for me: People do their best. I truly believe that, in most cases, if people could do better, they would. That includes me—forgiving myself is just as important as forgiving anyone else! Why don't people do better? We all have fears, hurts, insecurities, wounds, and unmet childhood needs that get in our way (big time!). Sometimes we just don't know better or we didn't learn better. Sometimes we do stuff just because we're stressed, hungry, or tired. The reason is not important. Compassion and understanding for the human condition is. Maybe your mom didn't love you the way you wanted her to love you. I believe she did her best. Maybe your spouse or partner doesn't always see you or hear you the way you want to be seen and heard. Can you believe they do their best? When you mess up, can you say to yourself, "If I could have done better, I would have done better"? Accept people's best, let go of the rest—that's what forgiveness is.

LESSON LEARNED

Forgiveness brings happiness and freedom. Carry with you a belief that people do their best. When you have compassion for what it means to be human, forgiveness comes easily.

Orange Ginger Glazed Salmon

Over the last few years I've had the pleasure of working with Sabrina Falone. She's an amazing food stylist and chef extraordinaire! This salmon recipe of hers proves it. It has an Asian flair and a fresh taste. It's also totally delicious and most definitely a meal you should serve to company. Thanks, Sabrina! Enjoy! **SERVES 4**

1. Preheat the oven to 425°F (220°C).
2. In a medium bowl, whisk together the orange zest, orange juice, cilantro (or green onion), ginger, sesame oil, and red pepper flakes (if using). Stir in half of the salt and half of the pepper. Set aside 2 Tbsp (30 mL) of this mixture (this will be used to glaze the top of the fish) then add the orange segments, red pepper, and snow peas and toss to combine. Let stand at room temperature for 15 minutes.
3. Meanwhile, arrange the salmon on a baking sheet lined with parchment paper. Season the top of each fillet with the remaining salt and pepper and brush with the reserved orange mixture. Bake for 10 to 15 minutes (depending on thickness of the fillets) or until the fish flakes easily with a fork.
4. To serve, spoon equal amounts of the marinated orange mixture over each fillet.

TIP

• Once the orange has been zested, you can segment it by slicing off the top and bottom to create two flat sides. Then run a sharp knife from top to bottom, following the shape of the orange, to remove the white pith; discard the pith. Using a paring knife, slice between each membrane to release the segments. Do this over a bowl to catch the fresh juice to use in the recipe.

PER SERVING (1 FILLET WITH ½ CUP/125 ML ORANGE MARINADE)
225 calories • 11 g fat • 2 g saturated fat • 8 g carbohydrates •
5 g sugars • 1.5 g fibre • 22 g protein • 352 mg sodium

Grated peel (zest) and segments from 1 navel orange

2 Tbsp (30 mL) orange juice

2 Tbsp (30 mL) finely chopped fresh cilantro leaves or green onion (white and green parts)

1 Tbsp (15 mL) minced gingerroot

2 tsp (10 mL) sesame oil

¼ tsp (1 mL) dried red pepper flakes (optional)

½ tsp (2.5 mL) salt, divided

½ tsp (2.5 mL) freshly ground black pepper, divided

½ cup (125 mL) thinly sliced red bell pepper

½ cup (125 mL) snow peas

4 salmon fillets (each about 3½ oz/100 g)

CONNECT WITH YOUR KIDS...
ANY WAY YOU CAN

> "To be in your children's memories tomorrow, you have to be in their lives today." **BARBARA JOHNSON**

How CONNECTED ARE you to your kids? Do you know how they are doing? Are they happy? Do they share with you their hopes, dreams, and fears? For me, some of the best connections I've had with my oldest daughter, Chelsea, have been via text messaging. Just about the time she was heading off to university she got a smart phone. Then I got one. Then we started to message each other. I was able to connect with her via her world (texting) as opposed to her connecting with me via mine. In my world connecting might mean the two of us going for a walk or sharing a cup of tea. In her world, this would be, well... boring! Anyway, via texting, my daughter and I got into a regular rhythm of conversation. This mode of communication worked well for her life and it worked well for mine, too. We often poked fun at each other, and we usually made each other laugh. I learned how to use all the little "emoticons," like happy faces, winking faces, and sticking out your tongue faces. And yet, among all the fun, I also managed to check in, see how she was doing, and always end with an "I love you!"

LESSON LEARNED

Staying connected to your kids and how they are doing is important. It doesn't matter how you connect. It only matters that you do.

Crumb-Topped Salmon with Parsley, Dill, and Lemon

How would you like a fast, easy, and totally delicious way to get more salmon into your family's diet? This recipe comes from Sylvia Kong, a food stylist from Calgary who I've had the pleasure to work with on multiple occasions. This recipe definitely gets two thumbs up—from both adults and kids. Thanks, Sylvia! Enjoy! **SERVES 4**

1. Preheat the oven to 425°F (220°C).
2. In a small bowl, combine the crumb topping ingredients. Set aside.
3. Arrange the salmon fillets on a baking sheet lined with parchment paper. Press equal amounts of the crumb topping evenly over the top of each fillet.
4. Bake for 10 to 15 minutes (depending on the thickness of the fillets) or until the fish flakes easily with a fork. Serve immediately.

TIPS

- For this recipe to be its best, use panko breadcrumbs. They are widely available at most supermarkets. Look for the whole-grain variety, but if they don't have it, buy the regular panko bread-crumbs (I will let you off the whole-grain hook just this once!). This type of crumb gives the fish an especially crispy topping.
- If you don't have fresh dill, you can substitute ⅛ tsp (0.5 mL) dried dill.
- The lemon crumb topping also works well on baked chicken breasts. I simply substitute an equal amount of fresh rosemary for the dill.

PER SERVING (1 FILLET) 262 calories · 14 g fat · 2.5 g saturated fat · 11 g carbohydrates · 0.6 g sugars · 2 g fibre · 23 g protein · 178 mg sodium

CRUMB TOPPING

⅔ cup (160 mL) whole-grain breadcrumbs

2 Tbsp (30 mL) extra virgin olive oil

1 Tbsp (15 mL) Dijon mustard

1 Tbsp (15 mL) light mayonnaise

2 Tbsp (30 mL) finely chopped fresh parsley leaves

1 tsp (5 mL) grated lemon peel (zest)

½ tsp (2.5 mL) finely chopped fresh dill

½ tsp (2.5 mL) freshly ground black pepper

FISH

4 salmon fillets (each about 3½ oz/100 g)

LIFE SHOULD BE JOYFUL!

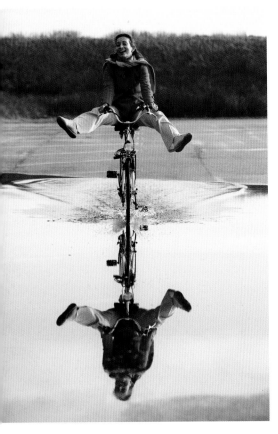

> "I define joy as a sustained sense of well-being and internal peace—a connection to what matters."
>
> **OPRAH WINFREY**

WHAT DOES THE word *joy* mean to you? To me joy is happiness on steroids. It's a feeling of sheer bliss. It's a sensation that life simply doesn't get any better. Here are just some of the things I link with joy:

- Falling in love/being in love
- Laughing so hard that I cry
- Working hard to achieve something really significant
- Time spent with friends I've known my whole life
- Listening to great music
- Dancing my heart out
- Singing my heart out
- Being totally silly and goofy
- Having a dream and making it happen
- Watching my kids feel joy
- Great food, good wine, a cold beer on a hot day... with friends
- Travelling the world
- Learning, reaching, discovering, growing
- Babies, puppies, kittens
- Witnessing greatness: a great speaker, a great show, a great athlete, a great movie
- Nature in all its magnificence
- Life
- What brings you joy?

LESSON LEARNED

Life should be joyful. Appreciate and cultivate the joy!

Rainbow Trout with Citrus, Ginger, and Fresh Thyme

Rainbow trout is loaded with disease-fighting omega-3 fats; low in mercury; and on the sustainable seafood list (which means it doesn't harm the environment or other fish and is not overfished). Quick and delicious this recipe deserves a place on your weekly menu. You can make it with any type of fish, including salmon or white fish. Enjoy! **SERVES 4**

1. Preheat the oven to 350°F (175°C).
2. In a small bowl, whisk together all of the marinade ingredients. Set aside.
3. Cut aluminum foil into four separate squares (each square must be large enough to totally wrap around and encase each fish fillet).
4. Arrange the foil squares on a baking sheet. Place each fillet onto the middle of a square.
5. Spoon the prepared marinade evenly over the top of each fillet. Fold the side of the foil up over the top of the fish and seal to make a tightly enclosed package (make sure it is fully sealed).
6. Transfer the baking sheet to the oven and bake for 7 to 12 minutes (depending on the thickness of the trout) or until the fish flakes easily when pierced with a fork.
7. To serve, gently remove the fish from the packets (be careful: the steam can burn you) and arrange on separate serving plates. Pour the juices over top each fillet and enjoy!

TIPS

- The fish and foil packets can be prepared several hours ahead and kept in the refrigerator until shortly before cooking.
- You can also cook the foil packets on your barbecue over medium heat.

PER SERVING (1 FILLET) 219 calories · 11.5 g fat · 2.5 g saturated fat · 8.4 g carbohydrates · 6 g sugars · 0.4 g fibre · 22 g protein · 189 mg sodium

MARINADE

½ cup (125 mL) orange juice

2 Tbsp (30 mL) freshly squeezed lemon juice

2 Tbsp (30 mL) minced gingerroot

1 Tbsp (15 mL) fresh thyme leaves

2 tsp (10 mL) liquid honey

1 tsp (5 mL) freshly grated lemon peel (zest)

2 cloves garlic, minced

2 jalapeño peppers, finely diced (seeds removed)

¼ tsp (1 mL) salt

¼ tsp (1 mL) freshly ground black pepper

FISH

4 rainbow trout fillets (each about 3½ oz/100 g)

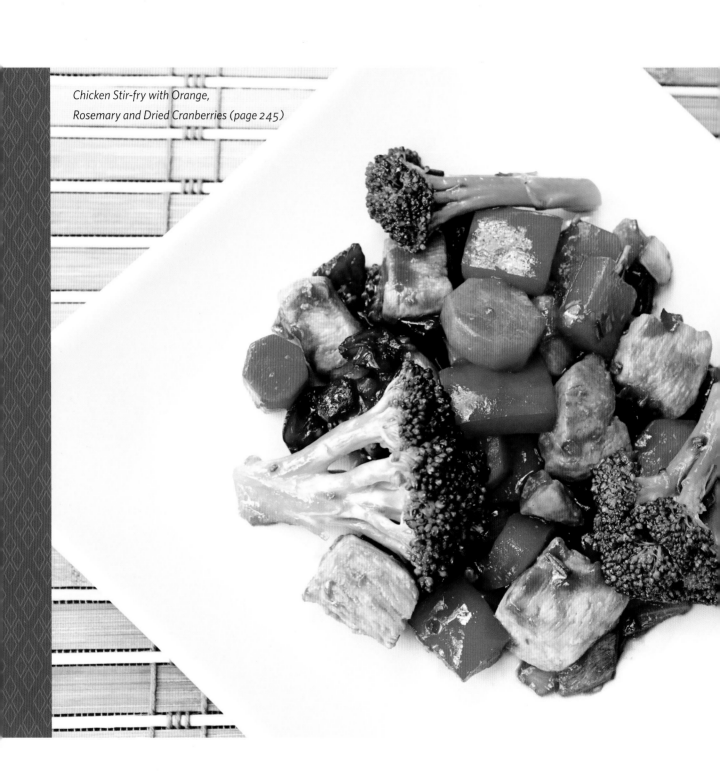

Chicken Stir-fry with Orange,
Rosemary and Dried Cranberries (page 245)

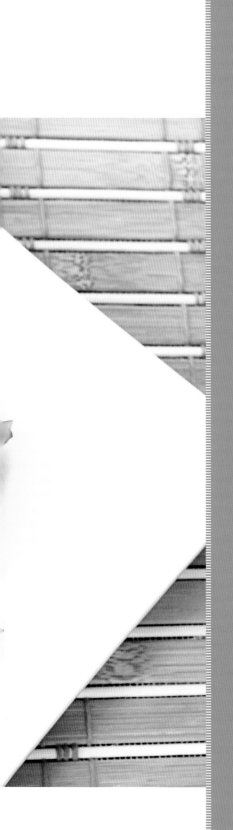

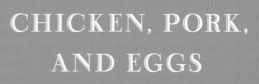

CHICKEN, PORK, AND EGGS

---

*A life lesson comes with
every recipe. Enjoy!*

IT'S A PRIVILEGE TO BE PART OF A TEAM

"A successful team beats with one heart." UNKNOWN

THREE YEARS AGO my neighbour invited me to play on a women's hockey team. I said yes, which is amusing for a number of reasons. First, the only time I'd ever played hockey was on a pond when I was a kid growing up, and I'd hardly call it hockey. Second, although I was a good skater, I'd never worn men's skates before, which are very different than women's figure skates. Third, I knew very little about the actual game of hockey, including basic rules like offside (which I got called on a lot in the beginning). Last, most of the women on the team were really good players! Luckily, these same women were also extremely patient with me (it helped that I am a quick learner and try really hard). I can tell you that today I really love the game of hockey and, more important, I've come to truly appreciate the beauty of a team. A team is so much more than people working together toward a common goal. It's also about friendship, support, camaraderie, fun, belonging, sharing, inspiration, and love. A team doesn't have to be sports-related. You and your spouse or partner can be one of the most beautiful teams there is. Your family can be an incredible team. Your neighbours can be a team. Most of us participate in teams in our work environment. Teams come in all shapes and sizes, and while it's important to be a good team player, I think it's equally important to appreciate the beauty of a team.

LESSON LEARNED

It is an honour and privilege to be part of a team. Don't take this honour for granted. What you gain and experience in the "togetherness" of a team simply can't be realized anywhere else.

Chicken Kebabs with Lemon, Oregano, and Fresh Parsley

If you love souvlaki, then you'll love this recipe. It's melt-in-your-mouth delicious and bursting with lemony flavour. You can serve it in whole-grain pita pockets or tortillas along with a bit of tzatziki, shredded lettuce, and tomato. It's also wonderful served alongside brown rice or quinoa and a green salad. Take any leftovers for lunch the next day—it's great hot or cold. Enjoy! **SERVES 4**

1. In a bowl, whisk together all of the marinade ingredients.
2. Add the chicken to the marinade and mix until well coated. Set aside for at least 15 minutes. (You can also cover and refrigerate overnight.)
3. Preheat the grill to medium heat.
4. Put the chicken on skewers. (If using wooden skewers, soak them first.)
5. Spray the grill with non-stick vegetable oil. Grill the chicken, turning every 2 minutes, for about 6 minutes or until cooked through. Serve and enjoy!

TIP
- This marinade also works wonderfully with pork, beef, or fish.

PER SERVING (1 SKEWER) 137 calories • 4 g fat • 1 g saturated fat • 2 g carbohydrates • 0.5 g sugars • 0.5 g fibre • 23 g protein • 195 mg sodium

MARINADE

1 green onion (white and green parts), chopped

Grated peel (zest) and juice of 1 lemon

½ cup (125 mL) finely chopped fresh parsley leaves

1 Tbsp (15 mL) extra virgin olive oil

1 tsp (5 mL) dried oregano leaves

2 cloves garlic, minced

¼ tsp (1 mL) salt

¼ tsp (1 mL) freshly ground black pepper

CHICKEN

14 oz (400 g) boneless, skinless chicken breasts (about 2 medium chicken breasts), trimmed of fat and cut into 1-inch (2.5 cm) cubes

WHAT'S YOUR BIG, GIANT, HAIRY GOAL?

"Don't bunt. Aim out of the ballpark."

DAVID OGILVY

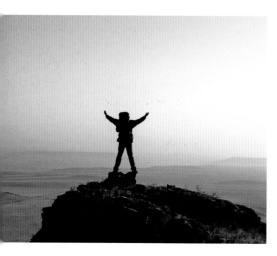

DO YOU SET goals? Do you wake up every day and have a list of all the things you want to get done? Do you plan your life for the next week, the next month, or even the next 10 years? Goal setting definitely keeps people on track. What really matters, however, is having big, giant, hairy goals. These are the kind of goals that drive you, excite you, and stir your soul. They're the kind of goals your heart aches for. What is your heart saying? How well do you listen? If you could do anything, be anything, and go anywhere, what would you choose? What would your life look like? Who would you be? Little, tiny, insignificant goals don't get you out of bed in the morning. Giant goals do. They ignite you. They pull you forward and keep you going, even when times get tough. Big, giant, hairy goals change your life and change who you are. Have the courage to set goals that are larger than life. Spend time with these goals. Make them so real that you can see, taste, and feel them before they even arrive. Let those goals drive you in the direction of your dreams.

LESSON LEARNED

Little goals don't drive you, excite you, or get you out of bed each day. Big, giant, oversized goals do. Let your big goals drive your little goals so that all your goals come true.

Chicken Stir-Fry with Basil, Cashews, and Peppers

Here's a quick and easy stir-fry that smells amazing, looks great, and tastes fantastic. It contains plenty of fresh, flavourful basil, and the cashews will please all the nut lovers. It makes a wonderful dinner, but the leftovers are great for lunch, too. Enjoy! **SERVES 4**

1. In a small bowl, whisk together the sauce ingredients. Set aside.
2. Heat a large frying pan or wok over medium heat. Spray with non-stick vegetable oil. Add the chicken and stir-fry until cooked and no longer pink inside, 4 to 6 minutes. Transfer the chicken to a plate and cover to keep warm.
3. In the same large frying pan or wok over medium heat, add the oil and onion and sauté until the onion is softened, 2 to 3 minutes Add the red pepper, jalapeño peppers, and cashews and sauté for another 3 minutes. Add the garlic and sauté for 30 seconds. Add the reserved chicken, prepared sauce, and basil. Stir-fry for about 2 minutes, making sure all the ingredients are well combined.
4. Serve with quinoa or whole-grain brown rice and a green salad.

TIPS

- If you'd prefer a spicier dish, add some of the seeds from the jalapeño peppers. The more seeds you add, the hotter it will be!
- For a lighter version of this dish, omit the cashews.

PER SERVING WITH CASHEWS (1 CUP/250 ML) 282 calories · 14.5 g fat · 2.5 g saturated fat · 12.5 g carbohydrates · 5 g sugars · 2.5 g fibre · 26 g protein · 335 mg sodium

PER SERVING WITHOUT CASHEWS (1 CUP/250 ML) 202 calories · 8 g fat · 1 g saturated fat · 9 g carbohydrates · 4 g sugars · 1.5 g fibre · 24 g protein · 316 mg sodium

SAUCE

2 Tbsp (30 mL) sodium-reduced soy sauce

1 Tbsp (15 mL) freshly squeezed lemon juice

1 tsp (5 mL) pure maple syrup

½ tsp (2.5 mL) cornstarch

STIR-FRY

14 oz (400 g) boneless, skinless chicken breasts (about 2 medium chicken breasts), cut into bite-size pieces

2 Tbsp (30 mL) extra virgin olive oil

1 onion, chopped

1 large red bell pepper, chopped

2 jalapeño peppers, finely chopped

¼ cup (60 mL) unsalted cashews (raw or roasted)

3 cloves garlic, minced

1 cup (250 mL) loosely packed chopped fresh basil leaves

THE SECRET TO LIVING YOUR DREAM LIFE

> "Poor is the man whose pleasures depend on the permission of another." **MADONNA**

WHAT'S STOPPING YOU from having the most incredible, awesome, wonderful life you can imagine? You. I believe most of us stop ourselves from getting what we want in life—love, happiness, a great job, financial abundance, and awesome relationships. Of course, we don't mean to do this. We're usually not even aware of the hundreds of ways we stop ourselves each day. It's the patterns we've learned, often since childhood. There is a voice inside us that tells us we are not capable or worthy of such a life. Patterns, however, can be changed. One way to change them is by giving ourselves permission to have the life that we want. It's simple, but very powerful. When you give yourself permission to live the life of your dreams, you open yourself up to receive that life. For example, I regularly give myself permission for the following:

- I give myself permission to fill my life with people who really love and care about me.
- I give myself permission to stand in my power and be all that I am capable of being.
- I give myself permission to be totally happy, joyful, and free.

Try it. Figure out what you want your life to look like. Give yourself permission every single day (repetition is important!) to have all that and more. Do it with feeling and conviction. Stand back and be amazed by what happens.

LESSON LEARNED

The person most responsible for stopping you from getting what you want in life is you. Don't sabotage your own happiness. Open yourself up to having a wonderful life by giving yourself permission to receive one.

Chicken Stir-Fry with Orange, Rosemary, and Dried Cranberries

Stir-fries are an awesome way to enjoy lean protein, like chicken breasts, along with a whole lot of vegetables. Enjoy them at home and when dining out. Teach your kids how to make them. This stir-fry is colourful, flavourful, and totally nutritious. Broccoli, red peppers, and carrots are all nutritional superstars, and dried cranberries are loaded with antioxidants. This stir-fry is also great warmed up for lunch the next day. **SERVES 4**

1. In a small bowl, whisk together the orange juice, soy sauce, cornstarch, and vinegar. Add the dried cranberries, rosemary, red pepper flakes, and garlic. Stir until combined. Set aside.

2. Heat a large frying pan or wok over medium heat. Spray with non-stick vegetable oil. Add the chicken and stir-fry until cooked and no longer pink inside, 4 to 6 minutes. Transfer the chicken to a plate and cover to keep warm.

3. In the same large frying pan or wok over medium heat, add the oil and onion. Sauté the onion for 2 to 3 minutes. Add the ginger, red pepper, broccoli, and carrots and stir-fry until the vegetables are tender-crisp, about 3 minutes. Add the prepared sauce and cooked chicken and continue stir-frying until the sauce thickens, about 2 minutes.

4. Serve with whole-grain brown rice or quinoa.

TIPS

- If you don't have fresh rosemary, substitute 2 tsp (10 mL) dried rosemary.
- If you'd prefer it spicy, add another ½ tsp (2.5 mL) of dried red pepper flakes to the sauce.
- For something different, try substituting ½ cup (125 mL) of fresh basil for the rosemary.

PER SERVING (1½ CUPS/375 ML) 302 calories ▪ 8.5 g fat ▪
1 g saturated fat ▪ 33 g carbohydrates ▪ 18 g sugars ▪ 4.5 g fibre ▪
27 g protein ▪ 386 mg sodium

SAUCE

½ cup (125 mL) orange juice

2 Tbsp (30 mL) sodium-reduced soy sauce

2 tsp (10 mL) cornstarch

2 tsp (10 mL) balsamic vinegar

½ cup (125 mL) dried cranberries

2 Tbsp (30 mL) chopped fresh rosemary leaves

½ tsp (2.5 mL) dried red pepper flakes

3 cloves garlic, minced

STIR-FRY

14 oz (400 g) boneless, skinless chicken breasts (about 2 medium chicken breasts)

2 Tbsp (30 mL) extra virgin olive oil

1 onion, chopped

1 Tbsp (15 mL) minced gingerroot

1 red bell pepper, chopped

1 large head of broccoli, chopped

3 carrots, chopped

THE NEED FOR HUMAN CONNECTION

"I define connection as the energy that exists between people when they feel seen, heard, and valued; when they can give and receive without judgment; and when they derive sustenance and strength from the relationship." **BRENÉ BROWN**

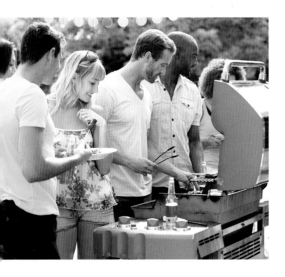

I BELIEVE THAT ALL human beings have a need to connect deeply with others. It is essential to our happiness and overall well-being. Connection happens when we are able to see, hear, feel, appreciate, or understand one another on some level. While connecting with family and friends is imperative to good health, life also presents endless opportunities to make connections with all those who cross your path each day. How often do you make the effort to truly connect with the bank teller, the waitress, or the cashier at the grocery store? Do you engage them in conversation? Do you make an effort to get to know who they are and what they are all about? When you make it your intention to connect with everyone you meet, many more connections take place. These small and frequent connections really make a difference. They make life more meaningful and more fulfilling. Don't underestimate their power. Smile. Ask questions. Say "Thank you" and "Have an awesome day!" Get good at connecting with everyone, everywhere you go. Your life (and their life!) will be so much richer for it.

LESSONS LEARNED

Never miss an opportunity to make a connection. By connecting to others, you connect to life and life connects to you.

Spiced Pork Tenderloin on the Grill

Pork tenderloin is one of the leanest cuts of meat you can eat. A healthy serving is about the size of a deck of cards. The spices in the marinade add great flavour and help to prevent carcinogens from forming when grilling. I made this for dinner recently and my daughter's friend said, "I love this! It has so much flavour and it's so moist." Enjoy! **SERVES 4**

1. In a medium bowl, whisk together all of the marinade ingredients. Set aside.
2. Using a sharp knife, trim the pork tenderloin of any fat and cut it lengthwise down the centre into two long strips.
3. Add the pork to the marinade. Turn to coat. Cover and refrigerate for at least 1 hour (or prepare it the day ahead and marinate overnight).
4. Preheat the grill to medium heat. Spray the grill with non-stick vegetable oil. Place the pork on the grill (discard the leftover marinade), close the lid, and cook 5 to 8 minutes per side, turning only once. Serve with grilled veggies or a green salad.

PER SERVING (3½ OZ/100 G) 167 calories • 2 g fat • 0.7 g saturated fat • 7 g carbohydrates • 0.5 g fibre • 21 g protein • 212 mg sodium

MARINADE

¼ cup (60 mL) orange juice

1 Tbsp (15 mL) sodium-reduced soy sauce

2 tsp (10 mL) pure maple syrup

1 tsp (5 mL) chili powder

1 tsp (5 mL) ground cinnamon

1 tsp (5 mL) ground cumin

1 Tbsp (15 mL) chopped fresh cilantro leaves

2 cloves fresh garlic, minced

MEAT

1 pork tenderloin (about 15 oz/450 g)

THREE SIMPLE WORDS WITH POWER BEYOND ALL OTHER

IMAGINE YOU ARE in a disagreement with someone you love. You are both trying to explain your point of view. You are both trying to justify your actions and tell your story. What if you dropped all the dialogue? What if you let go of the story? What if, instead, you took a deep breath, went inside your heart, and simply shared the following three words: *I love you.* These three simple words have power beyond all others. They are the most important words for us to hear and share. When walls don't allow other words to penetrate, these three words get through. They come from the heart, speak to the heart, and nourish the soul. *I love you.* Is there an opportunity for you to use these words more wisely? Do you realize how truly precious they are?

LESSON LEARNED

The most important words we can share with those we love are *I love you.* Don't get caught in a story when these three simple words will do.

One-Egg Omelette with Cremini Mushrooms, Basil, and Old Cheddar

A good friend of mine used to make this for me when I came to visit. It's delicious! I usually enjoy it for a quick lunch or dinner with a piece of whole-grain toast and a glass of milk. Double the ingredients if you want to share it with a friend. Omega-3 eggs are significantly higher in omega-3 fats, as well as vitamin E. Brown mushrooms, such as cremini, contain more antioxidants than white button mushrooms. For optimal taste, use the oldest cheddar you can find. Enjoy! **SERVES 1**

1. In a small non-stick frying pan over medium heat, heat the oil. Add the green onion and mushrooms and sauté until mushrooms are golden, 3 to 5 minutes.
2. Add the garlic, basil, and pepper and sauté for another minute. Transfer to a small bowl, cover, and keep warm. (Do not clean the frying pan.)
3. In the same frying pan, cook the egg over medium heat. Tilt and rotate the pan so the egg covers the bottom of the pan as it cooks. When the egg is almost set on the surface, carefully flip it to cook the other side.
4. Sprinkle half of the omelette with the cheese. Top with the reserved mushroom mixture. Fold the omelette in half over the mushrooms and slide onto a warm plate. Serve immediately.

PER SERVING (1 OMELETTE) 169 calories • 11 g fat • 3.5 g saturated fat • 4 g carbohydrates • 0.7 g fibre • 12 g protein • 169 mg sodium

1 tsp (5 mL) extra virgin olive oil

1 small green onion, chopped (white and green parts)

3 to 4 medium cremini mushrooms, sliced (about 1 cup/ 250 mL)

1 small clove garlic, minced

1 Tbsp (15 mL) chopped fresh basil leaves

¼ tsp (1 mL) freshly ground black pepper

1 large omega-3 egg, beaten

2 Tbsp (30 mL) shredded light old cheddar cheese

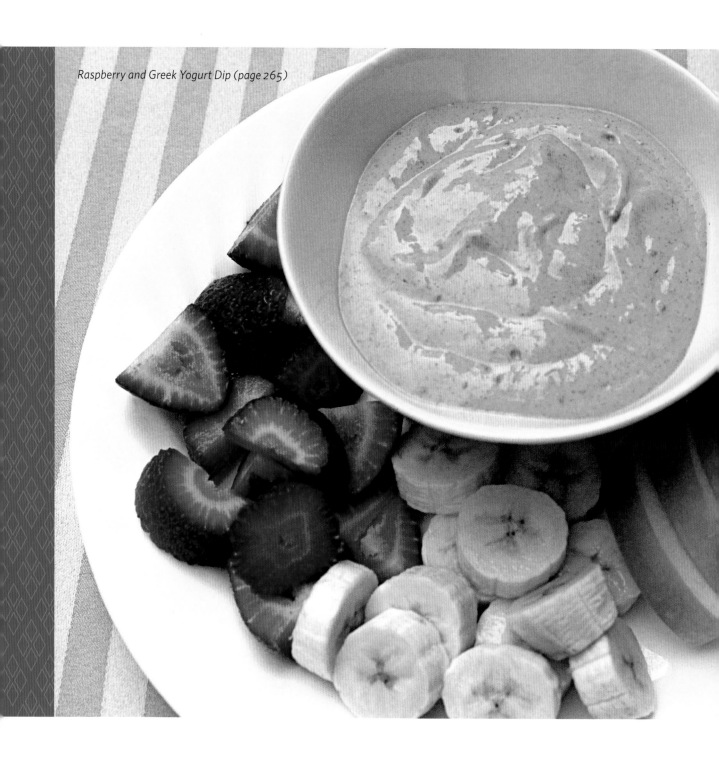

Raspberry and Greek Yogurt Dip (page 265)

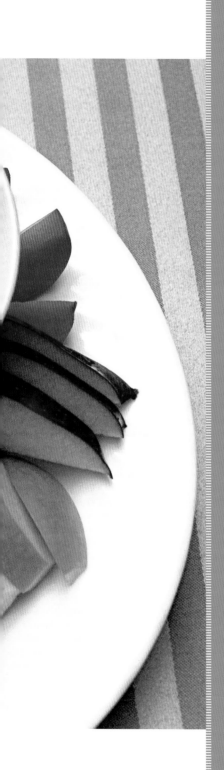

FUN AND HEALTHY SNACKS

*A life lesson comes with
every recipe. Enjoy!*

IF IT SCARES YOU, THEN DO IT

"You gain strength, courage, and confidence by every experience in which you really stop to look fear in the face. You must do the thing which you cannot do."

ELEANOR ROOSEVELT

I PLAY HOCKEY WITH a group of women on Friday nights. A men's team plays before us. Recently the men's team asked if any of the women could come out and play on Saturday night because they were short players. I agreed to play along with two other women. It was crazy! The players on the men's team were half our age. All of the players on the opposing team were men who could skate circles around us. I very courageously stayed on the ice for the whole game, even though I spent the entire time chasing the puck or avoiding slapshots that could kill someone. Would I play with them again? I don't think so. I did, however, flex my "do something every day that scares you" muscle. The only thing that holds you back in life is fear. The more things you do that are scary, the less scary life feels and the more willing you are to take on the next big challenge. The reverse is also true. If you avoid risk at every turn even the smallest risk can seem overwhelming. So flex your "take-a-risk" muscles. Each time a scary opportunity meets you along your journey, say to yourself, "Awesome! This must be the scary thing I'm supposed to do today!" Then go do it.

LESSON LEARNED
A great way to overcome fear is to regularly do things that scare you. Do something wonderfully scary today.

Super-Fresh Salsa

One of my girlfriends invited me to a euchre party with her co-workers. It was fun, even though I lost more games than I won. One of the guys at the party brought homemade salsa and tortilla chips. It was the freshest, most delicious salsa I've ever tasted. It put store-bought salsa to shame. His recipe inspired this recipe. Make sure you have a sharp knife for all the fine dicing. I suggest listening to some good salsa music while you are preparing this. I hope you enjoy this salsa as much as I do. Be sure to try it with Chili Lime Baked Tortilla Chips (page 261). **MAKES ABOUT 7 CUPS (1.75 L)**

1. Using a fine sieve, drain the juice from the diced tomatoes (discard the juice).
2. In a large bowl, combine all of the salsa ingredients, including the tomatoes. Set aside.
3. In a small bowl, whisk together the dressing ingredients. Drizzle the dressing over the salsa and mix well. Let sit for 4 hours at room temperature. Stir again, drain off the excess juice (if necessary), and serve.

TIPS

- If you want your salsa spicy, add some of the jalapeño seeds. The more seeds you add, the hotter it will be!
- Salsa also goes great with eggs, baked potatoes, fish, chicken, rice, quinoa, whole-grain crackers (such as Triscuit Thins), or whole-grain toast.

PER SERVING (½ CUP/125 ML) 36 calories • 2 g fat • 0.3 g saturated fat • 4 g carbohydrates • 2 g sugars • 1 g fibre • 0.8 g protein • 45 mg sodium

SALSA

4 cups (1 L) finely diced tomatoes (3 to 4 large tomatoes)

1 small onion, finely diced

1 small green bell pepper, finely diced

1 small red bell pepper, finely diced

2 jalapeño peppers (seeds removed), finely diced

1 bunch fresh cilantro leaves, chopped (about 1½ cups/ 375 mL, loosely packed)

DRESSING

2 Tbsp (30 mL) extra virgin olive oil

2 cloves garlic, minced

Grated peel (zest) and juice of 1 lime

½ tsp (2.5 mL) freshly ground black pepper

¼ tsp (1 mL) salt

THE MOST IMPORTANT LESSON FROM THE TRAGEDY OF 9/11

> "Love is life. And if you miss love, you miss life." **LEO BUSCAGLIA**

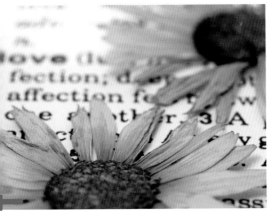

ON SEPTEMBER 11, 2001, the twin towers came down in New York City. Thousands of lives were lost. Minutes after the first tower was hit, more than 3,000 phone calls were made from people trapped inside the buildings. While some of the calls were pleas for help, most were to loved ones. In the final minutes, with death knocking at the door, people called their husband or wife, their mom and dad, their children and their best friends. What did they say? In phone call after phone call, the following three words: "I love you." What does this tell us? When death comes close, everything else falls away and love becomes the only thing that matters. We connect with who we are. We connect with what we feel. We connect with what's most significant in our lives. How connected are you to love right now? In your busy life, rushing here and there, doing this and that, do you still keep love at the forefront? Let the tragedy of 9/11 remind you of who you love most and what an incredible gift love is.

LESSON LEARNED

At the end of our lives many of us come to realize that what truly matters most is love. Don't wait until the end of your life to realize this truth. Live your life in love now.

Guacamole with Lime, Cumin, and Cilantro

Avocado is a nutritional powerhouse, rich in fibre, vitamin K, folate, and potassium. Although it's definitely not low in fat, the fat it contains is the good kind. This means that, in moderation, avocados definitely fit into a healthy diet. As for this recipe, my neighbour Mike said it was the best guacamole he'd tasted in his whole life. I'm not sure how many guacamole recipes Mike has tasted in his lifetime, but I do know that this recipe is pretty darn wonderful. I hope that you enjoy it as much as my neighbours and I do. Enjoy! **MAKES ABOUT 2½ CUPS (625 ML)**

1. In a medium bowl, using a fork, mash the avocados with the lime juice. Stir in the remaining ingredients.
2. Cover and refrigerate for about 30 minutes.
3. Serve with baked tortilla chips or whole-grain crackers.

TIPS

- If you'd like to add some kick to this dish, add some of the seeds from the jalapeño pepper. The more seeds you add, the hotter it will be!
- Sweet cocktail tomatoes are usually found in the produce department near the grape tomatoes and cherry tomatoes.

PER SERVING (½ CUP/125 ML) 107 calories • 9 g fat • 1 g saturated fat • 8 g carbohydrates • 2 g sugars • 5 g fibre • 2 g protein • 120 g sodium

2 avocados, mashed (about 2 cups/500 mL)

2 Tbsp (30 mL) freshly squeezed lime juice

1 cup (250 mL) diced sweet cocktail tomatoes

2 green onions (white and green parts), finely diced

1 jalapeño pepper (seeds removed), finely diced

2 cloves garlic, minced

¼ cup (60 mL) chopped fresh cilantro leaves

½ tsp (2.5 mL) ground cumin

¼ tsp (1 mL) salt

¼ tsp (1 mL) freshly ground black pepper

WHAT YOUR KIDS REALLY WANT

> "Even if society dictates that men and women should behave in certain ways, it is fathers and mothers who teach those ways to children—not just in the words they say, but in the lives they lead." **AUGUSTUS Y. NAPIER**

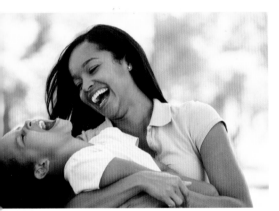

WHAT DO YOUR kids want and need from you the most? Without question, they want your love, your time, and your attention. They want to be seen, heard, and understood. They want to know that you care. What they also really want, however, is for you to be happy. Kids learn most not from what we say, but from what we do. When we are happy, we give our children permission to be happy. Are you a role model for happiness? Are you a role model for joy? Are you a role model for laughter, love, friendship, and living life well? The greatest gift we can give our children is to reach our full potential. They want to see us grow and learn and prosper. They want to see us thrive. When we don't thrive, our kids absorb our sadness, our broken dreams, and our lost hopes. They feel our pain. They don't know how to put a boundary between us and them. They absorb it all. Then they lug all our stuff around with them, often for a lifetime. Don't make your kids carry your un-lived life. Live a life you (and they) can be proud of. This doesn't mean that your kids should never see you cry or make mistakes. Life is also about tears and falling down. It just means that for the most part, your life is good. Are you living a good life?

LESSON LEARNED

One of the greatest gifts you can give your children is to be happy and live a great life. When you live your life well, you free your children to live their life well, too.

Dried Apricot and Greek Yogurt Hummus

How about a hummus dip that puts three powerhouse ingredients together? Chickpeas are a nutritional superstar; they're loaded with fibre, protein, folate, potassium, and iron. Greek yogurt gives you not only calcium, but an exceptional supply of protein, too. Dried apricots deliver much-needed potassium along with a powerful dose of antioxidants, including beta-carotene. They also add a touch of sweetness to this recipe that's just right. My neighbours (adults and kids) gave this hummus two thumbs up. Try it and let me know how many thumbs up you give it. Enjoy! **MAKES ABOUT 2 CUPS (500 ML)**

1. Place all of the ingredients in a food processor or blender and blend until smooth. If it's too thick, add up to ¼ cup (60 mL) water to adjust the consistency.
2. Serve immediately or refrigerate in an airtight container for up to 1 week. Enjoy with whole-grain crackers (like Triscuits), whole-grain pita bread, or cut-up veggies.

TIPS

- Do not add salt if you are using chickpeas that contain added salt.
- Tahini (sesame seed paste) is available at most large grocery stores and most health food stores. If you can't find it, ask.
- This hummus can also be made with dates instead of dried apricots. Try it both ways and let me know which one you prefer!

1 can (19 oz/540 mL) chickpeas (no salt added), drained and rinsed

½ cup (125 mL) plain low-fat Greek yogurt

¼ cup (60 mL) dried apricots

Grated peel (zest) of 1 lemon

¼ cup (60 mL) freshly squeezed lemon juice

2 Tbsp (30 mL) tahini (sesame seed paste)

2 cloves garlic

½ tsp (2.5 mL) ground cumin

¼ tsp (1 mL) freshly ground black pepper

¼ tsp (1 mL) salt

PER SERVING (¼ CUP/60 mL) 100 calories • 3 g fat • 0.5 g saturated fat • 13.5 g carbohydrates • 5.5 g sugars • 2 g fibre • 5 g protein • 87 mg sodium

GET COMFORTABLE WITH BEING UNCOMFORTABLE

> "Your life does not get better by chance, it gets better by change."
>
> **JIM ROHN**

How COMFORTABLE ARE you in your life right now? Chances are, if you're feeling really comfortable, you might be putting a limit on how beautiful your life can be. To learn, evolve, and grow we must change. The greater the growth, the greater the changes taking place. All change feels uncomfortable at first, even change that's good, because it's new and different. Do you embrace new and different? Are you willing to feel uncomfortable with new and different? Are you willing to change your relationships, your career, and who you are? Push yourself to get comfortable with what feels uncomfortable and then get uncomfortable again. Embrace the unknown. Take risks. Step beyond. Know that by pushing the boundaries of comfort, you push the boundaries of what your life can be.

LESSON LEARNED

Embrace the discomfort that comes with change. It's part of making your life all that you want it to be.

Black Bean and Chipotle Dip

Whenever I do television or media work in Calgary, I get the wonderful opportunity to work with Sylvia Kong. If I am demonstrating a recipe on a show like Breakfast Television, *Sylvia gets there before me and does the food styling and set-up of all the recipe ingredients. The last time I was in Calgary I asked her if she would be willing to contribute a couple of recipes to my next book. She most graciously said yes. I knew the recipes would be wonderful and, as always, Sylvia did not disappoint. This dip is super delicious and nutritious—black beans are a nutritional powerhouse. Thank you, Sylvia! Happy dipping!* **MAKES ABOUT 2 CUPS (500 ML)**

1 can (19 oz/540 mL) black beans (no sodium added), drained and rinsed

1 jalapeño pepper (seeds removed), chopped

¾ cup (185 mL) salsa

3 Tbsp (45 mL) freshly squeezed lime juice

2 Tbsp (30 mL) extra virgin olive oil

1 tsp (5 mL) chipotle chili powder

1 tsp (5 mL) ground cumin

1 clove garlic, minced

½ cup (125 mL) chopped fresh cilantro leaves

1. Using a blender (regular or hand-held) or food processor, blend all of the ingredients, except the cilantro, until smooth.
2. Transfer the bean mixture to a bowl and stir in the cilantro. Cover and refrigerate for at least 1 hour before serving. (Will keep, refrigerated, for up to 5 days.) Serve with tortilla chips or cut-up veggies.

TIPS

- If you prefer your dip on the spicy side, use hot salsa, rather than medium or mild, or leave in some of the seeds from the jalapeño pepper. The more seeds you add, the hotter it will be!
- The sodium content of salsa varies widely. Be sure to look for lower-sodium brands. You can always add a bit of extra salt if you really need to.

PER SERVING (¼ CUP/60 ML) 110 calories · 4 g fat · 0.5 g saturated fat · 15 g carbohydrates · 1 g sugars · 4 g fibre · 5 g protein · 95 g sodium

NOW THAT WAS A WONDERFUL HUG!

> "We need four hugs a day for survival. We need eight hugs a day for maintenance. We need twelve hugs a day for growth."
>
> **VIRGINIA SATIR**

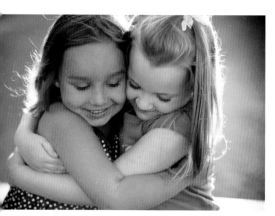

I DIDN'T GROW UP in a hugging family. As I've gotten older (and much wiser, of course), I've come to truly embrace the value of a great hug. Today I love getting, giving, or sharing a wonderful hug. Loving, physical touch is so important to our well-being. It nourishes our soul, touches our heart, and expresses deep emotion without the use of words. It softens our day. Do you express what you feel in the touch that you give? Do you use touch to say hello or goodbye or to help someone heal when they're hurting? Most important, do you know how to deliver a giant, all-encompassing, arms-fully-wrapped-around, squeezing-tight, love-filled hug? Why not give someone a hug like that today? Chances are they'll love it. And you'll love it, too!

LESSON LEARNED

Physical touch is essential to our well-being. Never underestimate the value of a great hug, both giving and receiving one. Great hugs are a beautiful part of life.

Chili Lime Baked Tortilla Chips

If you are going to have some chips with your dip, they should be healthy chips. Why not make your own? This recipe is fast and easy, and makes a fairly large batch. They have a subtle chili-lime flavour that both adults and kids will love. Be sure to buy 100% whole-grain flour tortillas, large size, and look for ones that are lower in sodium (the sodium content varies significantly from one brand to the next). Try these chips with Super-Fresh Salsa (page 253), Dried Apricot and Greek Yogurt Hummus (page 257), Guacamole with Lime, Cumin, and Cilantro (page 255), or Black Bean and Chipotle Dip (page 259). This recipe comes from Sylvia Kong, a food stylist in Calgary. She's amazing. Thanks, Sylvia! Enjoy!

MAKES 48 LARGE CHIPS

2 Tbsp (30 mL) freshly squeezed lime juice

1 Tbsp (15 mL) extra virgin olive oil

1 tsp (5 mL) chili powder

¼ tsp (1 mL) salt (optional)

6 large whole-grain soft flour tortillas

1. Preheat the oven to 375°F (190°C).
2. In a small bowl, whisk together the lime juice and oil. Set aside.
3. In another small bowl, combine the chili powder and salt.
4. Brush both sides of the tortillas with the lime mixture and then sprinkle with the chili mixture.
5. Stack the tortillas and, using a sharp knife, cut them into eighths to make chips (like cutting a pie). Arrange the tortilla wedges in a single layer on two baking sheets. Bake until golden and crisp, rotating the pans once. (The baking time will vary depending on the thickness of the tortillas. It may take anywhere from 7 to 15 minutes. Check frequently so they don't get too crisp.)
6. Let cool and store in an airtight container for up to 1 week.

PER SERVING (4 LARGE CHIPS MADE WITH ADDED SALT) 100 calories •
3.5 g fat • 0.6 g saturated fat • 15 g carbohydrates • 0 g sugars •
1.6 g fibre • 3 g protein • 177 mg sodium

PER SERVING (4 LARGE CHIPS MADE WITHOUT ADDED SALT) 100 calories •
3.5 g fat • 0.6 g saturated fat • 15 g carbohydrates • 0 g sugars •
1.6 g fibre • 3 g protein • 128 mg sodium

THE BEST WAY TO MOVE MOUNTAINS

> "Believe in yourself! Have faith in your abilities! Without a humble but reasonable confidence in your own powers you cannot be successful or happy."
>
> **NORMAN VINCENT PEALE**

THERE IS A song by Amanda Marshall called "I Believe In You." If you don't know the song, or even if you do, listen to it. Hear the words. Feel what they say. Appreciate their power. Do you have someone in your life who believes in you? Do you have someone who can prop you up and cheer you on when times get tough, when you need extra support, when you're wondering whether you're on the right path? Are you able to do this for yourself? When you experience self-doubt or question what you want or need or where you're going, can you say to yourself, "Don't worry, you'll figure it out. You can do this!" Don't ever underestimate the power of believing in yourself or others. Belief moves mountains and makes the impossible possible. Belief is the fuel for growth, change, and making dreams come true. Belief is everything! Believe in yourself. Believe in the people you love. Just believe!

LESSON LEARNED

Do your best to develop a rock-solid belief in yourself and others. It will fuel your dreams and theirs. Have incredible gratitude for those who believe in you.

Spinach and Greek Yogurt Dip with Fresh Basil

How would you like a dip that is loaded with great nutrition as well as flavour? Try this one. It's made with creamy, rich-tasting, protein-rich Greek yogurt. Spinach is, of course, a nutritional goldmine. The fresh basil and lemon put your taste buds into overdrive. My neighbour Linda said this dip is so good, it's addictive. Well, I guess if you're going to be addicted to something, it might as well be spinach dip! I like this dip served with 100% whole-grain Triscuit Thin Crisps crackers. They make an awesome combination. **MAKES ABOUT 3½ CUPS (875 ML)**

1. Using a blender (regular or hand-held) or food processor, blend all of the ingredients except the chopped basil until smooth.
2. Stir in the basil and serve with whole-grain crackers, cut-up veggies, or baked tortilla chips (page 261).

TIPS

- This recipe has no added salt. Taste it and add a pinch if you need to. If you serve it with salted crackers, however, you probably won't miss the salt.
- If you prefer, you can use about 8 cups (2 L) of fresh baby spinach instead of the frozen spinach. Frozen spinach is convenient and still offers outstanding nutrition.

2 cups (500 mL) low-fat plain Greek yogurt

1 package (10 oz/300 g) frozen chopped spinach, thawed and squeezed of excess water

2 cloves garlic, minced

1 Tbsp (15 mL) freshly squeezed lemon juice

1 Tbsp (15 mL) liquid honey

¼ tsp (1 mL) dried red pepper flakes

¼ tsp (1 mL) freshly ground black pepper

1 cup (250 mL) chopped fresh basil leaves

PER SERVING (½ CUP/125 ML) 66 calories • 2 g fat • 1 g saturated fat • 6 g carbohydrates • 4 g sugars • 1 g fibre • 8 g protein • 106 mg sodium

TAKE THE CEILING OFF FUN!

> "Today was good. Today was fun."
>
> **DR. SEUSS**

Last summer my daughter Shannon and five of her friends were playing in the park behind our house. It started to rain, so they all ran and took cover on our front porch. We watched as the rain poured down. All of a sudden my daughter runs off the porch and yells to her friends, "Come on, guys!" For the next half hour all six of them ran around in the pouring rain and got totally drenched. When Shannon finally came in to eat dinner and put on some warm clothes, she said, "That was so much fun!" So my question to you is this: How much fun are you having in your life right now? How many times a day do you laugh? How many times a day do you let yourself go a little crazy? Do you put a ceiling on the amount of fun you allow yourself to experience? What if there were no limit? What if one of your goals was to make life more fun? Having fun, each and every day, is one of my life goals. I look for fun and try to embrace it. I seek to lift the ceiling off fun or at least move the ceiling higher than it's been before. It's not always easy. Sometimes life gets in the way, but for the most part, I've found that when I look for fun, I'm much more likely to find and experience it. And guess what? Life becomes a lot more fun! How wonderful is that?

LESSON LEARNED

Life is way too short not to fill it with fun. Make fun a daily part of yours.

Raspberry and Greek Yogurt Dip

If you're going to serve a dip with a platter of fresh fruit, it might as well be nutritious. That way, you win twice. I want you to be a double winner! This dip, made with Greek yogurt and berries, is packed with good nutrition, including plenty of antioxidants, protein, and calcium. The cinnamon and lemon zest give it a real flavour kick. Enjoy!

MAKES ABOUT 3 CUPS (750 ML)

2 cups (500 mL) low-fat vanilla Greek yogurt

1 cup (250 mL) raspberries (fresh or frozen)

1 tsp (5 mL) ground cinnamon

1 tsp (5 mL) grated lemon peel (zest)

1. Using a blender (regular or hand-held) or food processor, blend all of the ingredients until smooth.
2. Serve with cut-up fresh fruit, such as strawberries, bananas, and apple slices.

TIPS

- You can substitute equal amounts of other berries, such as blueberries or strawberries, for the raspberries. Or try making three different dips, each with a different berry.
- Try this dip on top of fruit salad—it's wonderful!

PER SERVING (½ CUP/125 ML) 67 calories • 2 g fat • 1 g saturated fat • 7 g carbohydrates • 4 g sugars • 2 g fibre • 8 g protein • 46 g sodium

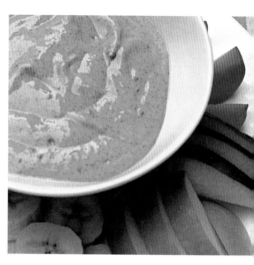

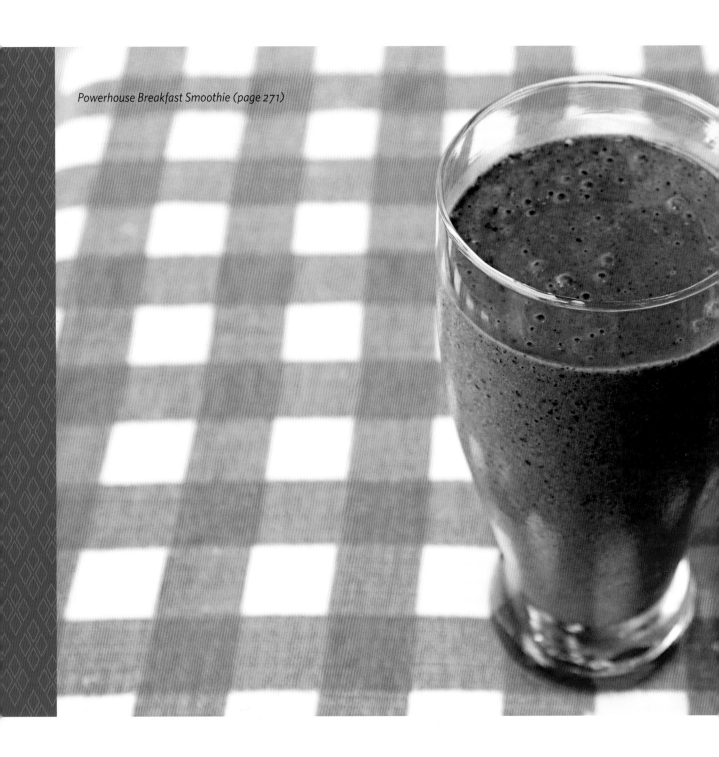

Powerhouse Breakfast Smoothie (page 271)

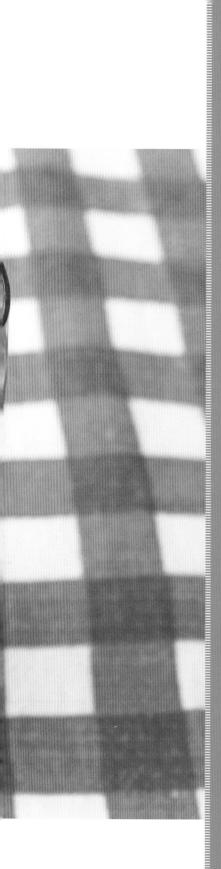

DRINKS AND SMOOTHIES

*A life lesson comes with
every recipe. Enjoy!*

CHERISH THE PEOPLE WHO LOVE YOU

> "Where there is love, there is life."
>
> **MAHATMA GANDHI**

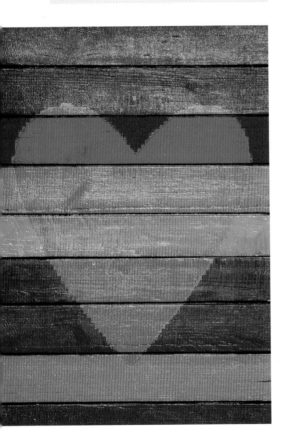

LOVE IS A gift. The older I get, the more I have come to understand and truly appreciate what a precious gift it is. Knowing this, I feel deep gratitude for all the people in my life who love me. When I say "all" the people, this includes members of my family, my neighbours, and my friends. It also includes people I meet on my travels each day who treat me with loving kindness. I cherish each and every one of them. The love they give feeds and sustains me. It makes my darkest days less dark and my sunniest days more brilliant. Love always makes life more beautiful and, most certainly, more meaningful, too. Are you aware of the people in your life who really love you? Do you cherish those people? Do you make time for them? Do you make every effort when they call or when you see them to love them back? Love is a gift—don't take the people who love you for granted.

LESSON LEARNED

There is nothing more wonderful, beautiful, meaningful, and valuable than love. Cherish the people who love you. They share with you a gift you simply can't get anywhere else.

Popeye's Favourite Smoothie

Here's a fun and delicious way to add some spinach to your life (plus it's loaded with great nutrition). Even your kids will love it, as long as they're okay with the colour green. If not, hunt down some old Popeye cartoons. Research shows that kids exposed to these cartoons eat more spinach. After all, if it's good for Popeye the Sailor Man, it must be good for them. Enjoy! **SERVES 4**

1. Using a blender (regular or hand-held), blend all of the ingredients until smooth.

   TIP
   - To freeze a banana, peel it first and then cut it into chunks. Place in a small resealable bag or container in the freezer until you are ready to use it.

   PER SERVING (1 CUP/250 ML) 129 calories · 1.5 g fat · 1 g saturated fat · 24 g carbohydrates · 16.5 g sugars · 2 g fibre · 6 g protein · 90 mg sodium

2 cups (500 mL) loosely packed baby spinach

1 cup (250 mL) low-fat milk (skim or 1%)

1 cup (250 mL) orange juice

½ cup (125 mL) low-fat vanilla Greek yogurt

1 cup (250 mL) strawberries (fresh or frozen)

1 medium banana, previously frozen in chunks

TWO WORDS THAT CAN TRULY CHANGE YOUR LIFE

> "No act of kindness, no matter how small, is ever wasted." **AESOP**

LIFE CAN SEEM so complicated at times. We wonder whether we'll ever figure things out. But things are often much simpler than we make them out to be. For example, there is incredible power in just two simple words: *kind* and *gentle*. These words can change your life if you let them. Don't be fooled by their simplicity. When you learn to be kind and gentle with yourself, your life transforms. When you learn to be kind and gentle with other people, their life transforms. We are all doing the best we can. We all make mistakes and fall down. We all get scared or do things we wish we'd done differently. The key is to be kind and gentle with yourself, and with others, through all of it. That's what real love looks like. It's kind and gentle. It doesn't yell or scream or expect us to be anything but what we are. Make every effort today and every day to be kind and gentle with yourself—in both words and actions—and to all those with whom you share life. It's an essential part of living life well.

LESSON LEARNED

Life can feel hard and complicated at times. One of the most powerful things you can do to make it easier is to be kind and gentle with yourself and others through all of it. It's a simple way to fill your life with love.

Powerhouse Breakfast Smoothie

Take three powerhouse superfoods—kale, mango, and wild blueberries—and combine them with soy milk and ginger. What have you got? A powerhouse smoothie that's fast, easy, and totally delicious. It's great for kids, too! Have it for breakfast or as a quick and easy mini-meal on the run. Your body will say thank you for sure. Enjoy! **SERVES 2**

1. Using a sharp knife, remove the thick rib that runs along the centre of each kale leaf and roughly chop the leaves (or use baby kale).
2. Using a blender, blend all of the ingredients until smooth.
3. Pour and serve.

TIPS
- I use frozen mango and blueberries because they're fast, convenient, and perfect for smoothies. Fresh fruit, however, is always an option.
- If you want extra fibre along with healthy omega-3 fats, add 1 to 2 tablespoons (15 to 30 mL) of ground flaxseeds.
- For a lighter version, use plain unsweetened soy milk or light strawberry soy milk, if available.

PER SERVING (1½ CUPS/375 ML) 234 calories · 4 g fat · 0.5 g saturated fat · 44 g carbohydrates · 30 g sugars · 6 g fibre · 9 g protein · 140 mg sodium

2 cups (500 mL) loosely packed chopped kale

2 cups (500 mL) strawberry soy milk

1 cup (250 mL) frozen mango cubes

1 cup (250 mL) frozen wild blueberries

One 1-inch (2.5 cm) piece gingerroot, sliced

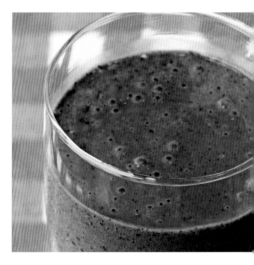

DARE TO LIVE IN THE GREY ZONE

MANY OF US think in terms of black and white. This is black and this is white. This is wrong and this is right. This is good and this is bad. This is why and this is why not. We have a point of view and we stick to it no matter what. Having an opinion is important, but you need to be very careful. If you want to be a student of life, you need to spend way more time in the grey zone. The grey zone is a place of questions and endless possibilities. What do we really know? Could we be wrong? What else haven't we thought about or considered? Could there be another way? Grey zone thinkers are thought leaders. They think and live outside the box and go places others dare not go. They're willing to say "I have no idea" and feel good about it. It can be uncomfortable and even scary to spend time in the grey zone. The wiser you become, however, the more likely it is that the grey zone becomes your home. You realize there is so much more you don't know than you do know. You become humble, and vulnerable. As a result, you learn and grow so much more than all the people who live in the black-and-white zone. Life as you know it expands.

"Be very, very patient and very open-minded, and listen to what people have to say." **A.J. MCLEAN**

LESSON LEARNED
Thinking only in terms of black and white limits our growth and ability to live life fully. Dare to live in the grey zone. Instead of giving answers, look for questions.

Spiced Cocoa Banana Smoothie

The cocoa bean from which cocoa and chocolate are made is loaded with plant compounds called flavanols. More and more research says these flava- nols protect health—they're good for your blood pressure, your heart, and your brain. This cold, frothy cocoa drink is a delicious and healthy way to get more cocoa into your daily diet. Enjoy!

P.S. The Kuna Indians, who are known for their healthy blood pres- sure and high cocoa consumption, also use bananas to sweeten their cocoa drinks. **MAKES 1 DRINK**

1. Using a blender (regular or hand-held), blend all of the ingredients until smooth.
2. Pour and serve.

TIP

- To freeze a banana, peel it first and then cut it into chunks. Place in a small resealable bag or container in the freezer until you are ready to use it.

PER DRINK 183 calories • 0.7 g fat • 0.2 g saturated fat • 38 g carbohydrates • 24 g sugars • 4.5 g fibre • 10 g protein • 104 mg sodium

1 cup (250 mL) low-fat milk (skim or 1%)

1 Tbsp (15 mL) natural unsweetened cocoa

1 frozen banana, cut into chunks

¼ tsp (1 mL) pure vanilla extract

¼ tsp (1 mL) ground nutmeg

¼ tsp (1 mL) ground cinnamon

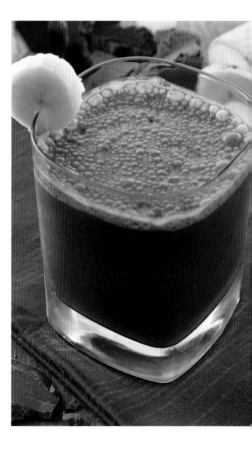

LOVE IS PATIENT AND LOVE IS KIND

"Never cut a tree down in the wintertime. Never make a negative decision in the low time. Never make your most important decisions when you are in your worst moods. Wait. Be patient. The storm will pass. The spring will come." **ROBERT SCHULLER**

I HAVE A CANVAS that hangs in the hallway of my house. It says "love is patient, love is kind". These are simple, but powerful words. Patience is defined as the ability to "bear or endure pain, difficulty, misfortune, provocation, or annoyance with fortitude and calm and without complaint." This is a fascinating definition. I never thought of patience as "enduring pain" and yet, patience and pain often go together. We experience pain when we sit in bad traffic or stand in a long line and especially when someone says or does something that makes us feel angry or hurt. If we practice patience, however, we handle that pain with "fortitude (courage) and calmness and without complaint". That's what love looks like. It means we don't get angry or anxious or mean, no matter what the situation. How patient are you? Are there people in your life (including you) or situations that you could be more patient with? Most importantly, are you willing to endure pain without complaint, knowing that ultimately this is the path to love?

How about kindness? "Love is kind." Kindness is defined by words like "caring, friendly, generous, helpful, courteous, considerate, and thoughtful." These are not selfish words. Do these words define you? Are there ways you could be more generous, more considerate, or more helpful to yourself or others? Kindness is also described as "not causing damage or harm." The people we often hurt most are the ones we are closest to (including ourselves). In what ways do your words or actions cause harm? Could you make choices that cause less? Most importantly, are you willing to practice kindness, knowing that this is the path to love?

LESSON LEARNED

If you want to master love, do your best to be master patience and kindness. That's what love is.

Chai Green Tea Vanilla Soy Latte

How would you like to add some pleasure to your day with a hot drink that's smooth, creamy, delightful, and also good for you? It's made with light vanilla soy milk, green tea, and spices. Soy milk is a nutritional powerhouse rich in protein, potassium, and magnesium along with added calcium, vitamin D, and vitamin B12. Like cow's milk, it contains a whole lot of nutrition in just one glass. The green tea and spices add great flavour as well as a healthy dose of antioxidants. This latte is a wonderful mid-morning or mid-afternoon drink. Enjoy! **MAKES 2 LATTES**

2 cups (500 mL) light vanilla soy milk

2 green tea bags

One 1-inch (2.5 cm) piece gingerroot, very thinly sliced

4 whole cinnamon sticks

6 whole cloves

¼ tsp (1 mL) ground cardamom

Freshly ground black pepper

1. In a small pot over low to medium heat, heat soy milk, green tea, ginger, and spices. As soon as the soy milk starts to boil, reduce the heat. Let it simmer gently for 5 minutes, stirring occasionally. Remove from the heat.

2. Using either a strainer or a slotted spoon, remove the cinnamon sticks, cloves, and ginger. Pour into mugs and enjoy!

TIP

• The advantage of using soy milk rather than regular milk (cow's milk) in this recipe is that you can simmer it and it won't separate.

PER SERVING (1 CUP/250 ML) 80 calories • 1.5 g fat • 0 g saturated fat • 7 g carbohydrates • 5 g sugars • 1 g fibre • 6 g protein • 110 mg sodium

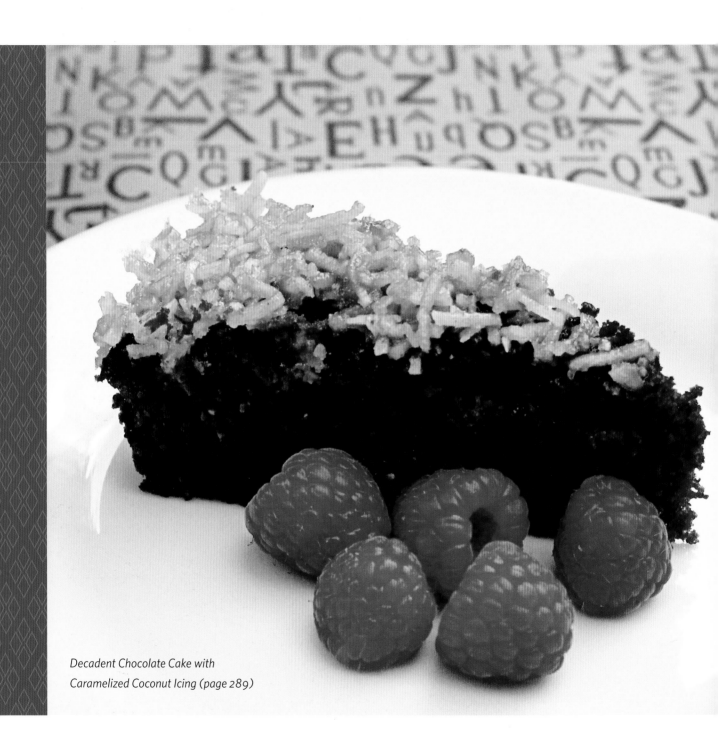

Decadent Chocolate Cake with
Caramelized Coconut Icing (page 289)

TREATS AND DESSERTS

Strawberries with Balsamic Vinegar,
Basil, and Lemon Zest *279*

Oatmeal Chocolate Chip Cookies with
Dried Apricots and Sunflower Seeds *281*

Chocolate Chip Cookies with Flax *283*

Oatmeal Berry Crisp with Lemon and Maple *285*

Maple Cinnamon Roasted Almonds *287*

Decadent Chocolate Cake with
Caramelized Coconut Icing *289*

*A life lesson comes with
every recipe. Enjoy!*

WHEN YOU SAY YES TO LIFE, THEN LIFE SAYS YES TO YOU

> "The big question is whether you are going to be able to say a hearty yes to your adventure."
>
> **JOSEPH CAMPBELL**

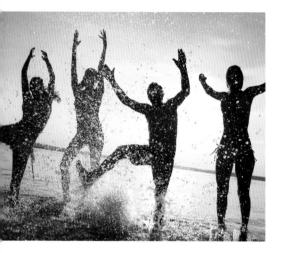

I HAVE MANY WONDERFUL neighbours. Linda is one of them. What I love about Linda is that she says YES to life. Her car is out of her driveway more often than it's parked. Dirty dishes left in her sink are not uncommon. Linda always has better things to do, other places to go, and good friends to visit. When Linda is home and I call her at the at the last minute to ask her to join me for a walk in the ravine or a beer in my backyard, more often than not she replies, "I'll be right over." Here's the important part of the story: Good things seem to happen for Linda. Some might say she's just lucky. I think it goes beyond that. I believe that when we say YES to life, then life responds by saying YES back. We get rewarded for living life well because that's the way life is meant to be lived. So here's the question: How good are you at saying YES to life? How well do you embrace the things, people, and places that make your heart sing? Is it possible that you could say YES more often?

LESSON LEARNED

When you embrace life and all that it has to offer, life responds in the affirmative. Be a person who says YES to life, so that life can say YES to you!

Strawberries with Balsamic Vinegar, Basil, and Lemon Zest

Berries are a superfood. Your body and your brain applaud you every time you eat them. Most often I enjoy my berries plain, just as they are. Sometimes, however, it's fun to dress them up, especially when you have company coming or want something a little more fancy. This recipe is fast, simple, and so fresh-tasting. Serve the berries along with a small scoop of low-fat frozen yogurt or a dollop of low-fat sour cream. Enjoy! **SERVES 4**

4 cups (1 L) chopped strawberries

¼ cup (60 mL) chopped fresh basil leaves

1 Tbsp (15 mL) balsamic vinegar

1 tsp (5 mL) pure maple syrup

½ tsp (2.5 mL) freshly grated lemon peel (zest)

¼ tsp (1 mL) freshly ground black pepper

1. In a medium bowl, combine the strawberries and basil.
2. In a small bowl, whisk together the remaining ingredients.
3. Add the vinegar mixture to the berry mixture and stir gently. Let sit at least 30 minutes before serving.

TIPS

- Try adding ½ tsp (2.5 mL) of cinnamon in Step 2 and let me know which version you prefer—with or without.
- You can use a combination of berries, including blueberries and raspberries, rather than simply strawberries (just know that strawberries and balsamic vinegar are an especially wonderful combination).

PER SERVING (1 CUP/250 ML) 60 calories • 0.5 g fat •
15 g carbohydrates • 10 g sugars • 3.5 g fibre • 1 g protein • 2 mg sodium

THE BEAUTY OF A BEST FRIEND

> "A single rose can be my garden... a single friend, my world."
>
> **LEO BUSCAGLIA**

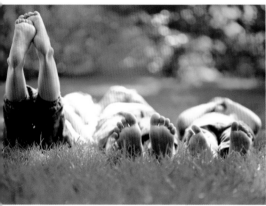

I GET SUCH TREMENDOUS joy from watching my youngest daughter, Shannon, and her best friend, Crysta. They have an incredibly special relationship, as all best friends do. They hang out together whenever they get the chance. They're always laughing about something, and often laughing hard. They try stuff as a pair that they might never try alone. They can be silly and goofy and crazy together, but also sad or grumpy. They love each other, care about each other, and are there for each other. These two girls are incredibly beautiful on their own, but as a unit their beauty is even bigger, bolder, and brighter. Do your best to cultivate and treasure the friends in your life, especially your best friends. There are few gifts that are as precious and life enhancing.

LESSON LEARNED

Best friends are meant to be cherished. They make life sweeter, brighter, and so much more beautiful.

Oatmeal Chocolate Chip Cookies with Dried Apricots and Sunflower Seeds

I love these cookies, but I don't make them very often. Why not? Because when I do, I eat them and often more than one! They're delicious, especially hot out of the oven along with a cold glass of milk. They're significantly better for you than your typical store-bought cookies, containing lots of good-for-you ingredients like whole-grain oats, dried apricots, and sunflower seeds. All cookies, however, should be enjoyed in moderation. Enjoy! **MAKES ABOUT 30 COOKIES**

½ cup (125 mL) soft-tub margarine

½ cup (125 mL) lightly packed brown sugar

1 omega-3 egg, beaten

1 tsp (5 mL) pure vanilla extract

1½ cups (375 mL) large-flake oats

½ cup (125 mL) whole-wheat flour

½ tsp (2.5 mL) baking soda

¼ cup (60 mL) unsalted sunflower seeds (raw or roasted)

¼ cup (60 mL) dried apricots, finely chopped

¼ cup (60 mL) dark chocolate chips

1. Preheat the oven to 350°F (175°C).
2. In a small bowl, cream together the margarine and brown sugar. Blend in the egg and vanilla. Set aside.
3. In a medium bowl, combine the oats, flour, and baking soda.
4. Add the small bowl of ingredients to the medium bowl of ingredients. Mix until just combined. Fold in the sunflower seeds, apricots, and chocolate chips.
5. Drop the dough by rounded teaspoons, about 2 inches (5 cm) apart, onto two baking sheets lined with parchment paper (about 15 cookies per sheet).
6. Bake for 7 to 8 minutes or until golden brown on the bottom but just barely cooked on top. Remove from the oven and let sit on the cookie sheet for another 5 minutes. Transfer the cookies to a rack to cool or enjoy right away.

TIPS
- Choose a margarine that is low in saturated fat and trans-fat-free.
- If you (or your kids) are not keen on having dried apricots or sunflower seeds in your cookies, this recipe can easily be made without them. They taste delicious either way!

PER COOKIE 84 calories • 5 g fat • 1 g saturated fat • 9 g carbohydrates • 4 g sugars • 1 g fibre • 0.8 g protein • 52 mg sodium

HAVE THE COURAGE TO GO OFF THE BEATEN PATH

> "Do not go where the path may lead, go instead where there is no path and leave a trail."
>
> **RALPH WALDO EMERSON**

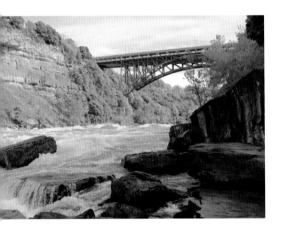

DURING MARCH BREAK I went on a two-day road trip to Niagara Falls with my youngest daughter, my sister, and her family. Although we participated in the expected tourist rituals, such as visiting the Falls, on day two of our trip we ventured off the beaten path. We drove along the Niagara River until we came to a cool lookout. From there, we climbed down a long, steep, slippery, rock-covered gorge to the river below. It was an exciting and sometimes treacherous journey, but one for which we were greatly rewarded. At the bottom we stood on a giant rock that jutted out over the water. The river itself was turquoise blue, powerful, pounding, and incredibly alive. The view was breathtaking. Magnificent memories are made and wonderful lessons learned when you travel off the beaten path. In fact, because each of us is so entirely unique, one could argue that the only way to truly live life well is to travel where others have not travelled before. Have the courage to live your life, at least some of the time, off the beaten path.

LESSON LEARNED

It can be challenging and takes courage to travel off the beaten path, but you often learn, grow, and experience so much more than those who travel only on the paths well worn by others.

Chocolate Chip Cookies with Flax

If you're going to have a cookie, why not have a cookie that tastes great but is made with healthier ingredients such as whole-wheat flour and ground flaxseeds? It's simply a better choice. Just remember that all cookies—even healthier ones—should be consumed in moderation. I suggest that once they come out of the oven you share them with friends or, once cooled, put them in an airtight container and limit yourself to just a cookie or two per day. Enjoy! **MAKES ABOUT 30 COOKIES**

½ cup (125 mL) soft-tub margarine

¾ cup (185 mL) lightly packed brown sugar

1 omega-3 egg, beaten

½ tsp (2.5 mL) pure vanilla extract

1 cup (250 mL) whole-wheat flour

¼ cup (60 mL) ground flaxseeds

½ tsp (2.5 mL) baking soda

⅓ cup (80 mL) dark chocolate chips or baking bits

1. Preheat the oven to 350°F (175°C).
2. In a small bowl, cream together the margarine and brown sugar. Blend in the egg and vanilla extract.
3. In a medium bowl, combine the flour, flaxseeds, and baking soda.
4. Add the small bowl of ingredients to the medium bowl of ingredients. Mix until just combined. Fold in the chocolate chips.
5. Drop the dough by rounded teaspoons, about 2 inches (5 cm) apart, onto two baking sheets lined with parchment paper (about 15 cookies per sheet).
6. Bake for 7 to 8 minutes or until golden brown on the bottom but just barely cooked on top. Remove from the oven and let sit on the cookie sheet for another 5 minutes. Transfer the cookies to a rack to cool or enjoy right away.

TIPS
- Choose a margarine that is low in saturated fat and trans-fat-free.
- You can buy flaxseeds pre-ground or grind them yourself with a clean coffee grinder.

PER COOKIE 73 calories • 4.5 g fat • 0.9 g saturated fat •
8 g carbohydrates • 5 g sugars • 0.5 g fibre • 1 g protein

A RECIPE FOR INSTANT JOY

> "Dance like there's nobody watching,
> Love like you'll never be hurt.
> Sing like there's nobody listening,
> And live like it's heaven on earth."
>
> **WILLIAM W. PURKEY**

I HAVE A RECIPE for instant joy. It really works! I hope you'll try it. Let's start with the ingredients. First we need you—amazing, fantastic, wonderful, beautiful you! Next we need some music, but not just any music. We need fabulous heart-pumping, soul-grabbing music that you love. Put the music on and turn it up loud. Now comes the fun part: Dance and sing your heart out. Do this in your living room or kitchen or wherever you want. You don't need a partner. In fact, by yourself is probably better because I want you to totally let go. Go crazy. Get into it. Be free. Sing. Dance. Twirl. Whatever! Then tell me how it feels. It certainly makes me feel great and always makes me smile. You may need to play your song more than once. The first time around may just be your warm-up. The main thing is to have fun, let loose, and truly enjoy yourself! Isn't that what life is for?

LESSON LEARNED

It's our job to create happiness and joy wherever we are. Spend some time singing and dancing today.

P.S. Your recipe for instant joy may be different than mine. That's okay. The most important thing is that you have one and use it often!

Oatmeal Berry Crisp with Lemon and Maple

I love this dessert! It also makes a great after-school snack. It's made with 100% whole-grain oats and loaded with antioxidant-rich, powerhouse berries. It's so delicious! It contains significantly less added sugar and fat than most traditional "crisp" recipes, and the fat it contains is the heart-healthy kind. The combination of spices, lemon zest, and maple syrup really brings the flavours to life. I hope you (and your kids) enjoy it as much as my family does. Enjoy! **SERVES 6 TO 8**

1. Preheat the oven to 375°F (190°C).
2. In a small bowl, combine the oats, brown sugar, nutmeg, and lemon zest. Cut the margarine into small cubes and add to the bowl. Using a fork, pastry blender, or potato masher, cut the margarine into the oatmeal mixture until crumbly. Set aside.
3. In a large bowl, combine the berries, flour, maple syrup, and cinnamon.
4. Transfer the berry mixture to an 8-inch (20 cm) square pan or baking dish. Sprinkle the oatmeal topping evenly over top.
5. Bake for 35 to 40 minutes or until the top is golden brown and the berry mixture is bubbling. Let cool for 5 to 10 minutes before serving.

TIPS

- Although you can use fresh or frozen berries in this recipe, I generally use frozen because they're so convenient and still loaded with great nutrition.
- Choose a margarine that is low in saturated fat and trans-fat-free.

PER SERVING (1 CUP/250 ML) 223 calories • 9 g fat • 1 g saturated fat • 34 g carbohydrates • 12 g sugars • 6.5 g fibre • 5 g protein • 60 mg sodium

CRISP TOPPING

1½ cups (375 mL) large-flake oats

⅓ cup (80 mL) lightly packed brown sugar

1 tsp (5 mL) ground nutmeg

Grated peel (zest) of 1 large lemon

¼ cup (60 mL) soft-tub margarine

BERRY BOTTOM

2 cups (500 mL) blueberries (fresh or frozen)

2 cups (500 mL) strawberries (fresh or frozen)

2 cups (500 mL) raspberries (fresh or frozen)

3 Tbsp (45 mL) whole-wheat flour

¼ cup (60 mL) pure maple syrup

1 Tbsp (15 mL) ground cinnamon

MAGIC HAPPENS WHEN YOU SAY GOODNIGHT WITH LOVE

"Sweet dreams, sleep tight, I love you, goodnight." **WORDS FROM A FRIEND**

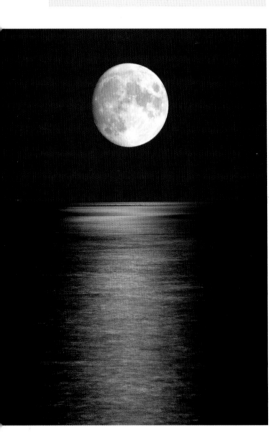

AT ONE TIME in my life I shared a relationship with a man who lived in another country. It was a long-distance romance. Long-distance relationships can be hard, and this one was, but it was also beautiful. It was here that I learned about the magic of saying goodnight with love. Each night just before I fell asleep, I received a goodnight email. No email was the same. Some were short and others long. Some spoke about what had taken place that day, while others were about the future or the past. All the emails, however, were beautiful, and all of them expressed love and gratitude ... love and gratitude for who I was, for what we shared, or for life in general. There is something so indescribable about falling asleep to words of genuine love and gratitude. There's no feeling like it. How well do you say goodnight to the people in your life? What words do you share with your spouse, your kids, or even yourself? Don't miss this opportunity. Take the time and make the effort. It is, without question, one of the most beautiful gifts you can give to another.

LESSON LEARNED

Few things in life are more beautiful than falling asleep to words of love and gratitude. Take time each night to express love and appreciation to the people who mean the most to you.

Maple Cinnamon Roasted Almonds

Almonds are the most nutrient-dense nut you can eat. They're especially rich in two disease-fighting nutrients most people don't get enough of: vitamin E and magnesium. We should all make an effort to eat a small handful of nuts every single day. Eating nuts plain, just as they are, is certainly the healthiest way to enjoy them, but a recipe like this one is a fun treat now and again. Your kids will love them, too! Enjoy! **SERVES 8**

2 cups (500 mL) unsalted raw whole almonds, skin on

3 Tbsp (45 mL) pure maple syrup

2 tsp (10 mL) canola oil

2 tsp (10 mL) pure vanilla extract

2 tsp (10 mL) ground cinnamon

1. Preheat the oven to 350°F (175°C).
2. Arrange the almonds in a single layer on a baking sheet and roast for about 10 minutes or until golden brown and fragrant. Remove from the oven and set aside.
3. Meanwhile, in a small saucepan over medium heat, combine the maple syrup, oil, vanilla, and cinnamon. Heat just until the mixture starts to boil. Remove from the heat.
4. Transfer the roasted almonds to the saucepan. Gently stir until the almonds are evenly glazed with the syrup mixture.
5. Line the same baking sheet with parchment paper and spray the paper with non-stick vegetable oil. Spread the maple almond mixture evenly onto the parchment paper and let cool.
6. Enjoy the same day or store in an airtight container in the refrigerator to nibble on throughout the week.

PER SERVING (¼ CUP/60 ML) 238 calories • 19 g fat • 1.5 g saturated fat • 13 g carbohydrates • 6 g sugars • 4.5 g fibre • 7.5 g protein • 1 mg sodium

HOW WELL DO YOU REALLY KNOW YOU?

> "A human being has so many skins inside, covering the depths of the heart. We know so many things, but we don't know ourselves! Why, thirty or forty skins or hides, as thick and hard as an ox's or bear's, cover the soul. Go into your own ground and learn to know yourself there."
>
> **MEISTER ECKHART**

LET'S SAY YOU'RE meeting a new friend for coffee. During your visit, how well would you get to know them? Would you talk about the weather or the daily news or would you talk about who they really are and who you really are? Would you want to get to know the deeper parts of them? Would you let them in to the deeper parts of you? How connected are you to what you feel, what you love most in life, your greatest fears and hurts, and your most significant shortfalls and strengths? Knowing yourself is so important! Make time each day to spend on your own in quiet reflection or meditation. Ask yourself: How am I feeling? What do I want and need? What makes me happy? Who am I, really? We don't ask these questions enough and yet the better we know ourselves, the greater our opportunity for happiness, authenticity, being truly comfortable in our own skin, and connecting to others. Just how happy, authentic, comfortable, and connected do you want to be? Are you devoting enough time to getting to know *you*?

LESSON LEARNED

When you become truly intimate with yourself, you open the door to true intimacy with others. That's why the best person to get to know well is yourself.

Decadent Chocolate Cake with Caramelized Coconut Icing

It's time for an awesome, decadent dessert. I am, after all, the dietitian who says "Leave room for chocolate!" This recipe comes from Lydia, a great friend and awesome cook. It's also the cake my daughters ask me to make on their birthdays. When I make it for guests, they always request the recipe. I've changed some of the ingredients to make the cake healthier than the original, but it's still not health food by any means and should be enjoyed on occasion and in small quantities. This cake truly gives new meaning to the word delicious. *If you make it once, it's highly likely you'll want to make it again and again. Enjoy!* **SERVES 12 SMALL PORTIONS OR 6 TO 8 MORE GENEROUS PORTIONS**

1. Preheat the oven to 350°F (175°C). Grease and flour one 9-inch (23 cm) round baking pan.
2. In a medium bowl, mix together the dry ingredients.
3. Add the wet ingredients to the dry ingredients and blend until smooth.
4. Pour the batter into the prepared baking pan. Bake for 20 to 25 minutes or until a toothpick inserted into the centre of the cake comes out clean.
5. Meanwhile, in a small bowl, combine the icing ingredients and stir until well mixed.
6. Spread the icing evenly over the warm cake. Turn the oven broiler on. Place the iced cake on the middle rack and broil until the top is bubbling and starting to turn golden brown, 3 to 5 minutes.
7. Remove from the oven and let cool. (You can also make it a day in advance.) Consider serving it with a scoop of light vanilla ice cream or frozen yogurt.

PER SERVING (WHEN CAKE IS CUT INTO 12 EVEN PIECES) 260 calories • 12 g fat • 3 g saturated fat • 37 g carbohydrates • 24 g sugars • 2.5 g fibre • 3 g protein • 133 mg sodium

DRY INGREDIENTS

1½ cups (375 mL) whole-wheat flour

¾ cup (185 mL) white sugar

3 Tbsp (45 mL) natural unsweetened cocoa

1 tsp (5 mL) baking soda

¼ tsp (1 mL) baking powder

WET INGREDIENTS

¼ cup (60 mL) canola oil

1 tsp (5 mL) white vinegar or cider vinegar

1 tsp (1 mL) pure vanilla extract

1 cup (1 mL) lukewarm water

ICING

¼ cup (60 mL) soft-tub margarine

½ cup (125 mL) lightly packed brown sugar

¾ cup (185 mL) sweetened shredded flaked coconut

1 Tbsp (15 mL) milk

Selected Bibliography

This bibliography includes some of the key research articles cited within each topic area. Not all studies are included due to the large number used. If you need further information on a particular study, contact me at liz@lizpearson.com.

SUPERFOODS

Abdull Razis, A., and Noor, N. "Cruciferous vegetables: dietary phytochemicals for cancer prevention." *Asian Pac J Cancer Prev.* 2013;14(3):1565–70.

Andújar, I., et al. "Cocoa polyphenols and their potential benefits for human health." *Oxid Med Cell Longev.* 2012;2012:906252.

Balakumar, P., and Taneja, G. "Fish oil and vascular endothelial protection: bench to bedside." *Free Radic Biol Med.* 2012 Jul 15;53(2):271–9.

Boyer, J., and Liu, R. "Apple phytochemicals and their health benefits." *Nutr J.* 2004 May 12;3;5.

Buitrago-Lopez, A., et al. "Chocolate consumption and cardiometabolic disorders: systematic review and meta-analysis." *BMJ.* 2011 Aug 26;343:d4488.

Carlsen, M., et al. "The total antioxidant content of more than 3,100 foods, beverages, spices, herbs, and supplements used worldwide." *Nutr J.* 2010 Jan 22;9:3.

Cartea, M., et al. "Phenolic compounds in Brassica vegetables." *Molecules.* 2010 Dec 30;16(1):251–80.

Darmadi-Blackberry, I. "Legumes: the most important dietary predictor of survival in older people of different ethnicities." *Asia Pac J Clin Nutr.* 2004; 13 (2):217–20.

Desideri, G., et al. "Benefits in cognitive function, blood pressure, and insulin resistance through cocoa flavanol consumption in elderly subjects with mild cognitive impairment: the Cocoa, Cognition, and Aging (CoCoA) study." *Hypertension.* 2012 Sep;60(3):794–801.

Dhingra, D., et al. "Dietary fibre in foods: a review." *J Food Sci Technol.* 2012 Jun;49(3):255–66.

Drewnowski, A., "The Nutrient Rich Foods Index helps to identify healthy, affordable foods." *Am J Clin Nutr.* 2010 Apr;91(4):1095S–1101S.

Flores-Mateo, G., et al. "Nut intake and adiposity: meta-analysis of clinical trials." *Am J Clin Nutr.* 2013 Jun;97(6):1346–55.

Giacalone, M., et al. "Antioxidant and neuroprotective properties of blueberry polyphenols: a critical review." *Nutr Neurosci.* 2011 May;14(3):119–25.

Hegarty, B., and Parker, G. "Fish oil as a management component for mood disorders—an evolving signal." *Curr Opin Psychiatry.* 2013 Jan;26(1):33–40.

Hollenberg, N., et al. "Flavanols, the Kuna, cocoa consumption, and nitric oxide." *J Am Soc Hypertens.* 2009 Mar–Apr;3(2):105–12.

Hooper, L., et al. "Effects of chocolate, cocoa, and flavan-3-ols on cardiovascular health: a systematic review and meta-analysis of randomized trials." *Am J Clin Nutr.* 2012 Mar;95(3):740–51.

Hyson, D.A. "A comprehensive review of apples and apple components and their relationship to human health." *Adv Nutr.* 2011 Sep;2(5):408–20.

Jonnalagadda, S., et al. "Putting the whole-grain puzzle together: health benefits associated with whole grains—summary of American Society for Nutrition 2010 Satellite Symposium." *J Nutr.* 2011 May;141(5):1011S–22S.

Jungbauer, A., and Medjakovic, S. "Anti-inflammatory properties of culinary herbs and spices that ameliorate the effects of metabolic syndrome." *Maturitas.* 2012 Mar;71(3):227–39.

Kapusta-Duch, J., et al. "The beneficial effects of Brassica vegetables on human health." *Rocz Panstw Zakl Hig.* 2012;63(4):389–95.

Katz, D., et al. "Cocoa and chocolate in human health and disease." *Antioxid Redox Signal.* 2011 Nov 15;15(10):2779–811.

Khan, N., and Mukhtar, H. "Tea and health: studies in humans." *Curr Pharm Des.* 2013;19(34):6141–7.

Kromhout, D. "Omega-3 fatty acids and coronary heart disease: the final verdict?" *Curr Opin Lipidol.* 2012 Dec;23(6):554–9.

Martín-Peláez, S., et al. "Health effects of olive oil polyphenols: recent advances and possibilities for the use of health claims." *Mol Nutr Food Res.* 2013 May;57(5):760–71.

Mitchell, D., et al. "Consumption of dry beans, peas, and lentils could improve diet quality in the US population." *J Am Diet Assoc.* 2009 May;109(5):909–13.

Panickar, K. "Beneficial effects of herbs, spices, and medicinal plants on the metabolic syndrome, brain, and cognitive function." *Cent Nerv Syst Agents Med Chem.* 2013 Mar;13(1):13–29.

Papanikolaou, Y., and Fulgoni, V. "Bean consumption is associated with greater nutrient intake, reduced systolic blood pressure, lower body weight, and a smaller waist circumference in adults: results from the National Health and Nutrition Examination Survey 1999–2002." *J Am Coll Nutr.* 2008 Oct;27(5):569–76.

Ras, R., et al. "Tea consumption enhances endothelial-dependent vasodilation: a meta-analysis." *PLoS One.* 2011 Mar 4;6(3):e16974.

Sabaté, J., and Ang, Y. "Nuts and health outcomes: new epidemiologic evidence." *Am J Clin Nutr.* 2009 May;89(5):1643S–1648S.

Siriwardhana, N., et al. "Health benefits of n-3 polyunsaturated fatty acids: eicosapentaenoic acid and docosahexaenoic acid." *Adv Food Nutr Res.* 2012;65:211–22.

Tighe, P., et al. "Effect of increased consumption of whole-grain foods on blood pressure and other cardiovascular risk markers in healthy middle-aged persons: a randomized controlled trial." *Am J Clin Nutr.* 2010 Oct;92(4):733–40.

Yang, C., and Hong, J. "Prevention of chronic diseases by tea: possible mechanisms and human relevance." *Annu Rev Nutr.* 2013;33:161–81.

DIETARY VILLAINS AND OTHER HEALTH HAZARDS

Aburto, N., et al. "Effect of lower sodium intake on health: systematic review and meta-analyses." *BMJ.* 2013 Apr 3; 346:f1326.

Bauer, K., et al. "Parental employment and work–family stress: associations with family food environments." *Soc Sci Med.* 2012 Aug;7(3):496–504.

Basu, S. "The relationship of sugar to population-level diabetes prevalence: an econometric analysis of repeated cross-sectional data." *PLoS One.* 2013;8(2):e57873.

Bray, G., and Popkin, B. "Calorie-sweetened beverages and fructose: what have we learned 10 years later." *Pediatr Obes.* 2013 Aug;8(4):242–8.

Duffey, K., and Popkin, B. "Energy density, portion size, and eating occasions: contributions to increased energy intake in the United States, 1977–2006." *PLoS Med.* 2011 Jun;8(6):e1001050.

Gallimberti, L. "Energy drink consumption in children and early adolescents." *Eur J Pediatr.* 2013 Oct;172(10):1335–40.

Garcia, G., et al. "The fast food and obesity link: consumption patterns and severity of obesity." *Obes Surg.* 2012 May;22 (5):810–8.

George, E., et al. "Chronic disease and sitting time in middle-aged Australian males: findings from the 45 and Up study." *Int J Behav Nutr Phys Act.* 2013 Feb 8;10:20.

Gunja, N., and Brown, J. "Energy drinks: health risks and toxicity." *Med J Aust.* 2012 Jan 16;196(1):46–9.

He, F. "Effect of longer-term modest salt reduction on blood pressure." *Cochrane Database Syst Rev.* 2013 Apr 30;4:CD004937.

Kruger, J., et al. "Dietary practices, dining out behavior, and physical activity correlates of weight loss maintenance." *Prev Chronic Dis.* 2008 Jan;5(1):A11.

Lachat, C., et al. "Eating out of home and its association with dietary intake: a systematic review of the evidence." *Obes Rev.* 2012 Apr;13(4):329–46.

Marshall, B., and Levy S. "Food animals and antimicrobials: impacts on human health." *Clin Microbiol Rev.* 2011 Oct;24(4):718–33.

Powell, L., and Nguyen, B. "Fast-food and full-service restaurant consumption among children and adolescents: effect on energy, beverage, and nutrient intake." *JAMA Pediatr.* 2013 Jan;167(1):14–20.

Rippe, J., and Angelopoulos, T. "Sucrose, high-fructose corn syrup, and fructose, their metabolism and potential health effects: what do we really know?" *Adv Nutr.* 2013 Mar 1;4(2):236–45.

Rohrmann, S. "Meat consumption and mortality—results from the European Prospective Investigation into Cancer and Nutrition." *BMC Med.* 2013 Mar 7;11:63.

Santarelli, R., et al. "Processed meat and colorectal cancer: a review of epidemiologic and experimental evidence." *Nutr Cancer.* 2008;60(2):131–44.

Stanhope, K., et al. "Adverse metabolic effects of dietary fructose: results from the recent epidemiological, clinical, and mechanistic studies." *Curr Opin Lipidol.* 2013 Jun;24(3):198–206.

Van der Ploeg, H., et al. "Sitting time and all-cause mortality risk in 222,497 Australian adults." *Arch Intern Med.* 2012 Mar 26;172(6):494–500.

Van Horn, L., et al. "Translation and implementation of added sugars consumption recommendations: a conference report from the American Heart Association Added Sugars Conference 2010." *Circulation.* 2010 Dec 7;122(23):2470–90.

Willet, W. "Dietary fats and coronary heart disease." *J Intern Med.* 2012 Jul;272(1):13–24.

Wolk, B., et al. "Toxicity of energy drinks." *Curr Opin Pediatr.* 2012 Apr;24(2):243–51.

QUESTIONS THAT NEED ANSWERS

Ben-Shoshan, M. "Vitamin D deficiency/insufficiency and challenges in developing global vitamin D fortification and supplementation policy in adults." *Int J Vitam Nutr Res.* 2012 Aug;82(4):237–59.

Bischoff-Ferrari, H., et al. "A pooled analysis of vitamin D dose requirements for fracture prevention." *N Engl J Med.* 2012 Jul 5;367(1):40–9.

Brien, S., et al. "Effect of alcohol consumption on biological markers associated with risk of coronary heart disease: systematic review and meta-analysis of interventional studies." *BMJ,* 2011;342(feb22 1):d636.

Fedirko, V., et al. "Alcohol drinking and colorectal cancer risk: an overall and dose-response meta-analysis of published studies." *Ann Oncol.* 2011 Sep;22(9):1958–72.

Gaziano, J., et al. "Multivitamins in the prevention of cancer in men: the Physicians' Health Study II randomized controlled trial." *JAMA.* 2012 Nov 14;308(18):1871–80.

Hemilä, H., and Chalker, E. "Vitamin C for preventing and treating the common cold." *Cochrane Database Syst Rev.* 2013 Jan 31;1:CD000980.

Huang, H., et al. "Multivitamin/mineral supplements and prevention of chronic disease." *Evid Rep Technol Assess* (Full Rep). 2006 May;(139):1–117.

Ma, Y., et al. "Association between vitamin D and risk of colorectal cancer: a systematic review of prospective studies." *J Clin Oncol.* 2011 Oct 1; 29(28):3775–82.

Michaëlsson, K., et al. "Long-term calcium intake and rates of all cause and cardiovascular mortality: Community-based prospective longitudinal cohort study." *BMJ.* 2013 Feb 12;346:f228.

Nair, R., and Maseeh, A. "Vitamin D: The 'sunshine' vitamin." *J Pharmacol Pharmacother.* 2012 Apr;3(2):118–26.

Nelson, D., et al. "Alcohol-attributable cancer deaths and years of potential life lost in the United States." *Am J Public Health.* 2013 Apr;103(4):641–8.

Poli, A., et al. "Moderate alcohol use and health: a consensus paper." *Nutr Metab Cardiovasc Dis.* 2013 Apr 30. S0939-4753(13)00067-7.

Popkin, B., et al. "Water, hydration and health." *Nutr Rev.* 2010 August; 68(8):439–458.

Rice, B., et al. "Meeting and exceeding dairy recommendations: effects of dairy consumption on nutrient intakes and risk of chronic disease." *Nutr Rev.* 2013 Apr;71(4):209–23.

Rong, Y., et al. "Egg consumption and risk of coronary heart disease and stroke: dose-response meta-analysis of prospective cohort studies." *BMJ.* 2013 Jan 7;346:e8539.

Ronksley, P., et al. "Association of alcohol consumption with selected cardiovascular disease outcomes: a systematic review and meta-analysis." *BMJ,* 2011;342(feb22 1):d671.

Schöttker, B. "Strong associations of 25-hydroxyvitamin D concentrations with all-cause, cardiovascular, cancer, and respiratory disease mortality in a large cohort study." *Am J Clin Nutr.* 2013 Apr;97(4):782–93.

MAKING SENSE OF FOOD MYTHS AND MISUNDERSTANDINGS

Freedman, N., et al. "Association of coffee drinking with total and cause-specific mortality." *N Engl J Med.* 2012 May 17;366(20):1891–904.

Grover, S., et al. "Probiotics for human health—new innovations and emerging trends." *Gut Pathog.* 2012 Nov 26;4(1):15.

Jirillo, E. "Healthy effects exerted by prebiotics, probiotics, and symbiotics with special reference to their impact on the immune system." *Int J Vitam Nutr Res.* 2012 Jun;82(3):200–8.

Lee, A., et al. "The effect of substituting alternative grains in the diet on the nutritional profile of the gluten-free diet." *J Hum Nutr Diet.* 2009 Aug;22(4): 359–63.

Li, G., et al. "Coffee consumption and risk of colorectal cancer: a meta-analysis of observational studies." *Public Health Nutr.* 2013 Feb;16(2):346–57.

Sanz, Y. "Effects of a gluten-free diet on gut microbiota and immune function in healthy adult humans." *Gut Microbes.* 2010 May–Jun;1(3):135–7.

Simpson, S., and Thompson, T. "Nutrition assessment in celiac disease." *Gastrointest Endosc Clin N Am.* 2012 Oct;22(4):797–809.

Smith-Spangler, C. "Are organic foods safer or healthier than conventional alternatives?: a systematic review." *Ann Intern Med.* 2012 Sep 4;157(5):348–66.

LOSING WEIGHT, KEEPING IT OFF, AND STAYING ACTIVE

Chaput, J., and Tremblay, A. "Adequate sleep to improve the treatment of obesity." *CMAJ.* 2012 Dec 11;184(18):1975–6.

Chen, L., et al. "Reduction in consumption of sugar-sweetened beverages is associated with weight loss: the PREMIER trial." *Am J Clin Nutr.* 2009 May;89(5):1299–306.

Dansinger, M., et al. "Comparison of the Atkins, Ornish, Weight Watchers, and Zone diets for weight loss and heart disease risk reduction: a randomized trial." *JAMA.* 2005 Jan 5;293(1):43–53.

Hargens, T, et al. "Association between sleep disorders, obesity, and exercise: a review." *Nat Sci Sleep.* 2013 Mar 1;5:27–35.

Jakicic, J., et al. "American College of Sports Medicine position stand. Appropriate intervention strategies for weight loss and prevention of weight regain for adults." *Med Sci Sports Exerc.* 2001 Dec;33(12):2145–56.

Kaipainen, K., et al. "Mindless eating challenge: retention, weight outcomes, and barriers for changes in a public web-based healthy eating and weight loss program." *J Med Internet Res.* 2012 Dec 17;14(6):e168.

Tremblay, M., et al. "New Canadian physical activity guidelines." *Appl Physiol Nutr Metab.* 2011 Feb;36(1):36–46; 47–58.

Wilmot, E., et al. "Sedentary time in adults and the association with diabetes, cardiovascular disease, and death: systematic review and meta-analysis." *Diabetologia.* 2012 Nov;55(11):2895–905.

Nutrition Index

dark chocolate, 44, 45
milk chocolate, 44, 45
white chocolate, 44
chocolate milk, 53, 87–88
cholesterol, 54, 92, 93, 125
LDL cholesterol, 9, 23, 29, 32, 103, 108
HDL cholesterol, 9, 32, 60, 75
citrus fruit and juice, 83, 91, 98, 99, 100, 106
coconut
coconut milk, 85
coconut oil, 34
coconut water, 91
coffee, 42, 53, 59, 61, 64, 65, 87, 89, 91, 102, 107–109
constipation, 22, 29, 30, 89, 110, 111
crackers, 27, 28, 105, 106
cruciferous vegetables, 11–13, 98

D

dark leafy greens, 7, 14–16, 49, 55, 83, 85, 98
DASH diet, 99
dementia, 6, 7, 17, 18, 23, 31, 32, 35, 36, 40, 41, 44, 60, 75, 76, 78, 90, 107, 124
dental health, 7, 40, 59, 66, 86, 91
depression, 35, 36, 37, 38, 74, 78, 79, 84, 99, 107, 123
diabetes, 11, 18, 19, 20, 22, 23, 26, 30, 40, 43, 48, 54, 59, 63, 64, 67, 69, 75, 78, 86, 92, 93, 99, 100, 107, 110, 114, 122, 123, 125
dining out, 48–53, 57, 71, 78, 120
buffet restaurants, 51
fast food, 48, 49, 50, 51, 52, 53, 57, 58, 71, 103, 120
dried fruit, 30, 52, 61, 62, 98, 105, 106

E

eating on the run, 49
eating out, *see dining out*

eggs, 92–94
energy drinks, 59, 61, 65–66
eye health, 14, 19, 37, 82, 83, 92

F

fat, 14–15, 19, 31, 32, 37, 38, 45, 49, 53, 70, 71, 87, 92, 109, 119
omega-3 fats, 20, 31, 35–39, 94
healthy fats, 31, 48, 92
unhealthy fats, 31, 32, 49, 76, 92, 109, 111
fast food, *see dining out*
fibre, 9, 19, 22, 25, 26, 28, 29–30, 81, 83, 99, 102, 106, 111, 114
fish, 31, 35–39, 52, 58, 69, 71, 80, 92
contaminants, 37
fish oil capsules, 37, 38
mercury, 37, 39, 112
salmon, 35, 38, 39, 80, 93
shellfish, 38, 93
tuna, 39, 58
flavonoids, 17, 20, 25, 40, 42
flavanols, 43
flaxseeds, 20, 21, 29, 30, 93, 94
food labels, 27, 28, 30, 39, 57, 60, 61
food portions, 8, 10, 12, 16, 20, 23, 33, 38, 42, 45, 51, 52, 53, 68, 71, 86, 119
free radicals, 6, 7, 9, 11, 33, 41, 44, 107
frozen dinners, 58
fruit, 30, 48, 49, 51, 55, 60, 61, 66, 81, 92, 98–101, 103, 105, 106, 111, 113, 120, 121
fruit juice, 89, 100

G

gallstones, 19, 89, 107
garlic, 17, 70
gastrointestinal health, 10, 22, 29, 30, 69, 110–112, 113–114
genes, 8, 11, 33, 41, 68, 100
genetically modified food, 100–101
gluten-free, 28, 113–114
gout, 59, 63, 86, 107

granola bars, 59, 60, 106
grapes, 7, 98

H

hearing loss, 37
heart disease, 6, 7, 9, 11, 14, 17, 18, 19, 21, 22, 23, 26, 29, 30, 31, 32, 35, 36, 38, 40, 43, 45, 48, 49, 54, 55, 59–60, 67, 68–69, 70, 75, 76, 78, 79, 81, 82, 85, 86, 92, 93, 98, 99, 107–108, 110, 112, 114, 122, 126
herbs and spices, 17–18, 42, 58, 62, 69, 70, 91
high blood pressure, 9, 21, 23, 26, 29, 43, 44, 54, 55, 56, 59, 63, 74, 99, 120, 122, 125
high blood sugar, 11, 23, 27–28, 29, 44, 54, 66, 75, 86, 89, 107, 122, 123, 126

I

ice cream, 59, 87
immunity, 6, 7, 12, 17, 29, 31, 37, 40, 41, 74, 78, 81, 83, 110, 122, 123
inflammation, 6, 9, 12, 17, 18, 19, 23, 25, 30, 31, 32, 33, 35, 36, 40, 43, 54, 59, 68, 75, 107, 108, 113, 114, 123–124
inflammatory bowel disease, 30, 31–32, 110
iron, *see vitamins and minerals*

K

kale, 11–13, 14–16, 98
kidney health
kidney disease, 90
kidney failure, 55
kidney stones, 56, 63, 64, 80, 82, 83, 86, 99
kiwi, 83, 98, 99

L

lactose intolerance, 86, 110
legumes, *see beans*
lignans, 20

Recipe Index

About the Author

LIZ PEARSON, RD, is a registered dietitian with a passion for peanut butter sandwiches and an undying love for chocolate. She also loves to dance! Liz is the author of three books, including *The Ultimate Healthy Eating Plan (That Still Leaves Room for Chocolate)* and *Ultimate Foods for Ultimate Health (And Don't Forget the Chocolate!)*. Her last two books were national bestsellers and both won awards of excellence, including the Gold Award from Cuisine Canada, which celebrates superior food writing and recipes. Liz was the "Ask the Expert" nutrition columnist for *Chatelaine* magazine for almost seven years. She appears regularly on radio and television across Canada, including CityTV's *Breakfast Television* and CBC radio. As a professional speaker, Liz is asked to speak frequently to corporations, associations, and health professionals about food, life, and living well. She is a regular consultant to the food industry, including companies such as Loblaws, Catelli, and Nestlé. Last, but certainly not least, Liz has two daughters and lives in Toronto. Liz believes that "food, love, and life should be delicious!" Her mission is to make your life more so!

P.S. Check out Liz's website at www.lizpearson.com and be sure to subscribe to her blog when you're there.